Angling Therapy

Note: the speckled trout (Cynoscion nebulosus) on the cover was photographed by the author and released to spawn.

Visit www.booksurge.com to order additional copies.

Angling Therapy

James Michael Doggett

2007

Angling Therapy

Whom the gods would destroy
They first make a bonefisherman.

—-Van Campen Heilner, author, angler, and alleged alcoholic,1935(I).

For Mom and Dad, and every American Soldier, Sailor and Airman for giving me the chance to fish marine waters around the world, and to safely return home to the greatest nation on the planet.
—- Jim Doggett, West Galveston Bay, Texas, U.S.A.
March 5th, 2007

RICK

THIS WILL ALWAYS BE A MAGIC HOUR, I thought to myself. Not dawn. The magic happens an hour or so after that. With the sun's climbing angle in a cloudless sky, the early morning glare on the water's surface, that liquid mirror like quicksilver that shields everything beneath from a hunter's eye, quickly vanishes. A slight change in angle and, suddenly, sunlight penetrates into the water instead of reflects, and the light creates a window through which I may once again gaze into an alien world on earth. And here before me, revealed like a new gift to a child—even when given to this child day after day for years on end—was, inarguably, America's most seductive and challenging marine hunting ground, the Florida Keys: translucent, emerald green water covers the white coral sand bottom of natural channels that course an intricate, seemingly endless, glowing path through lush beds of submerged turtle grass that are a darker lime rind green. These beds and channels stretch for miles, paralleling and criss-crossing the chain of islands, extending outward to the east on a ledge of coral limestone and marl to living coral reefs of the Atlantic shelf , and to the west over the sand, mud and marl of the more drainage sediment-base of the Everglades, Florida Bay and finally the clear Gulf of Mexico. At some of the keys the sea grass beds taper up to shallower white and ochre sand and mud flats, and, finally, beach; at the meeting with other keys, grass beds and sand suddenly plunge to form deep and dark, undercut banks that are shadowed by overhanging mangrove branches and leaves, the rusty red, barnacle encrusted roots of which extend down into the dark, sheltered water like a reaper's long, twisted fingers. In these shadows lurk any number of creatures, most of them on the hunt, all of them on the hiding because, as in all food chains where life begins with the light of the sun, there will always be one more species of prey than there is predator. But this does not take into account the ultimate predator that always wins: time.

It was the channels that my guide, Captain Rick Miller, and I concentrated our eyes on. Illuminated now, reflecting the translucent green of plankton, we would easily be able to see the dark, blue-green backs of migrating tarpon contrasting over the white bottom. Once the sun is high the fish stand out almost as starkly as black exclamation points on a piece of white paper. It is a highly visual game, and in late spring and early summer when the tarpon migrate, it can last a length of time that mirrors a working man's work day of eight hours, throughout which, if the sky is clear, the visibility into the water is good in at least one direction or another for spotting fish from the height of a boat, until the sun begins to take on too steep an angle to the western horizon for even the best polarized lens to penetrate through the water. The glare returns and the window closes. Time wins again.

Although concentrating on, and into, the water immediately before us, flashes of light a half mile away on the water's surface nonetheless drew my eye. There, in the white channel that paralleled the broken shoreline of Key Largo, were hundreds of white sunburst flashes, each of them occurring as sunlight bounced off a tarpon's silver head and following iridescent back as she rolled above the surface of the water, like a dolphin, and briefly entered our world to breathe in the same ambient air that Rick and I breathed. There were so many fish in the school, each of them a briefly flashing star, that they created a counter-flowing current of water that stretched for more than a hundred yards behind them on the flat surface of the inshore Atlantic.

I quietly watched them for a minute or two before I finally pointed my twelve weight fly rod to the school of fish, turned to look at Rick on the poling platform above the outboard and said, "That's such a strength— breathing air, but it's also their undoing."

I had interrupted my guide's own private reverie. He smiled and said, "If they tasted good it surely would be." It is a rare luxury in sight fishing, time is. Too much of it can allow "performance anxiety" to root itself into the psyche of an insecure angler. Rick and I were beyond that, as individual anglers and as a team. What we got out of it, each time the inevitable moment approached, was a focused adrenalin, a controlled anticipation and a near-giddiness that is a realization, a physical manifestation and proof to each of us that there is no better game in the world, and that we are ready for it once again. It is a confident state of ecstasy that is the product, the reward, of the single-minded obsession of the athlete. The fish drew closer, but were still several minutes away, rolling happily like children at play time.

Tarpon, *Megalops atlanticus* (the taxonomic genus and species of identification; here, in Greek: "big-eyed of the Atlantic"), more ancient than terrestrial dinosaurs in their origin, yet still extant and virtually unchanged, have a highly vascularized swim bladder, a buoyancy organ like a submarine's ballast tanks that, in the tarpon's case, does double duty by serving as a functional lung to supplement the oxygen they glean from water through their gills. It allows them to survive in oxygen-depleted waters throughout their youth, where there are fewer predators, those mostly birds. Tarpon must breathe air as adults, too, and thereby announce themselves with every breath to the world of Man. But if they know they are being hunted from above, they can hold their breath for a long time and survive on gill-oxygen. A pragmatic "scientist" once put a few great fish in a completely filled and lidded, though highly oxygenated water tank; all tarpon were dead within a couple of days (2, Cole).

The tarpon before us now, still undisturbed, continued up the channel, as it cut a comfortable and familiar path for them across the shallower sea grass beds, a path they had taken for eons on their annual migration, a path that changed only marginally as shape-shifting storms and ice ages reoriented it from time to time. Although there was enough water for them to swim directly across the sea grass, tarpon seem to love following channels: they are like fish highways, and the entire length of a channel's edge with sea grass beds does provide excellent ambush hunting habitat, like a long, nearly endless buffet. As the channel reached a jutting peninsula that marked the end of the Key Largo cove we faced, it swung out abruptly in a hairpin turn and upon reaching it, the tarpon seemed to hesitate for a moment before regrouping, turning with it and continuing along its path, probably remembering this course change in their migratory microchip minds. They were heading due east now in the green channel, into the sun, straight along their trek to where Rick and I awaited them on his cleverly positioned skiff, where I stood like a heron at the ready on the casting platform with fly and rod in hand.

They were now only a hundred yards away, closing at the pace of a brisk walk.

I knew I would be the first thing to interrupt the day of these peaceful fish.

We could hear them breathing now, more than a hundred rushing sighs that rose slowly and progressively in volume as they approached. I was reminded of a big herd of horses. Two hundred feet away, and the sound of their breathing had now grown to fill our ears and shut out thought of anything else. A brooding unease settled in my chest. It was an atavistic sense that something was wrong, that something *BIG* was going to happen: there were just too many big fish, too much wild game, too concentrated in one small, albeit moving, spot. There was a palpable feeling of massive, collective energy restrained but unquestionably hair-triggered. *Stick to routine.* I looked at my feet on the deck, at the loose coils of fly line that I had stripped off my fly reel and stowed out of wind's way in the cockpit. No tangles. This is comforting, Standard Operating Procedure of the saltwater angler. A quick glance to my guide on the poling platform: Rick looked flat-out suspicious; while concentrating on the fish ahead of us, he made a quick little glance to our ocean-side, as if there were something watching *us*, something just outside this scene of reserved calm.

When the lead tarpon—and there were at least four or five of them at the head of this massive school that was as wide as the channel itself, some ninety feet—rolled and broke the surface one hundred and twenty feet off the bow, I could see the black outline of their inordinately large eyes actually above the water for an instant, and then the blue-black iridescence of the scales on their backs. They were all good-sized fish, on either side of six-feet and a hundred pounds, but I picked out my target fish to lead, a fish in the center, and roll-cast the rod forward; this created a loop of energy in the fly line that plucked the orange grizzly tarpon fly from my pinched left thumb and index finger, and this energy directed out forward pulled more fly line out of the rod guides and loaded it nicely for the back cast, and as I began it, my left hand—my line hand—had now been freed of the fly and smoothly switched over to grip the fly line that had been tucked beneath my right index finger to the rod handle, for uninterrupted line control. I brought the rod back, bending it with the momentum of the aerialized fly line, simultaneously hauling on the fly line in the opposite direction, and then released the tension in the line with the line hand and let it shoot out behind me before catching it again for more momentum to load the rod for the fore cast, and after one more cycle I was ready now, four seconds into the cast, to make my presentation of the fly to the lead fish, which is what this whole game is all about really, putting a fly in front of a fish, a fish which was at present one hundred feet away. Right as I shot the cast out to the fish, the line on the deck at my feet now jumping up into the air and zipping through the rod guides on its journey to connect us together, angler and fish, a dark gray dorsal fin some three or four feet in height above the surface of the Atlantic inshore water screamed into my field of view from the left, the ocean side, impossibly fast, into the edge of the school, and the emerald green water of the channel directly in front of us, and the calm water over the sea grass beds in every direction around us, all instantaneously exploded up into the air and outward under water, all roared in a foaming white pandemonium. It was violence, wild pure violence, everything roaring in water and rattling in air, and up through the water to our ears was transmitted a tearing, gnashing, ripping thunderclap of tumult that lasted a whole of three to five seconds.

Then nothing but calm. There was a blossomed plume of copper colored water out in front of the becalmed skiff where a tarpon had been bitten very roughly in half.

"Great Hammerhead," Rick said.

I couldn't say anything yet.

"Breakfast, I guess. Now we know why so many fish were together and they were so calm—they hadn't been hit yet, not today, not for a while, anyway."

My brain played catch-up: The shark had come in from a paralleling channel separated from the school's channel by a dense grove of sea grass beds in roughly three feet of water that had helped to break up his form, his pattern, probably even his wake somewhat, until the last minute when he'd hopped over the beds at full speed for a side intercept into the school. Ambush. He was every bit as big as Rick's seventeen foot skiff. That something so large could move so quickly, so fast as to appear to me as merely a huge gray-brown blur of motion, was more than unsettling; it was as if I had witnessed a *perversion* of nature not meant to be seen. But it was the norm, and it happened every day for tarpon and shark.

We stood quietly for a long moment, Rick on his tall platform, I on the front of his skiff with my fly rod, now held impotently in a slack hand. My heart slowed down from its double-dose of adrenalin. "Thanks," I said aloud.

"Me?" Rick asked, after a moment's hesitation.

"Yes, you," I said, looking at him "For allowing me to see all this. Everything. Thanks."

He shook his head. "That was straight from the hand of God, Jim. But you're welcome."

* * *

It was the first hammerhead attack on migratory tarpon I had ever witnessed. I would learn that, more from guides and my own observations than from my university marine biology studies, some populations of the Great Hammerhead, _Sphyrna mokarran_, follow the tarpon throughout their migration, picking them up here and there, in a constantly unfolding event seasonally driven by latitudinal changes in water temperature, availability and migrations of their respective prey, and the optimum conditions for breeding in a defining predator and prey relationship that has its roots back in the Jurassic period, some one hundred and thirty five million years past (3, Bond).

I was humbled, there on my guide's modern skiff, and not by any lack of grace I may have had with a fly rod. This visual world had been given to me on a silver platter simply because I was doing what I wanted to do, the one thing that made me feel whole again. And what an honor: Rick had invited me to be his angler, his weapon of choice, in the twenty-ninth annual Gold Cup Tarpon Tournament, the most historically significant invitational fly tourney in the world, entirely free of charge. I can assure you it wasn't because of any gratuity to Rick which, though he said mine was overly generous at twenty percent, he announced that tips never made for a good day on the water. At four hundred dollars per day, even back then, in 1992, Rick's was a rare gift indeed. I gave his offer about three second's worth of stunned thought: two days of exploratory fishing and five days of fishing a world-renowned tournament, all for free. Hmmm....I was a little concerned about possibly tainting the higher calling of angling with competition, but I would try and refrain from any judgment until after I had at least tried it myself. And besides, the Gold Cup was started, in the very year I was born, by the greatest hitter that ever lived, Ted Williams, the Splendid Splinter, a man who also answered the call to duty as a fighter pilot when war interrupted his baseball career. It is no oddity to me that he was also an excellent fly caster and angler, and hid out in Islamorada in the off-season to chase these same fish with his guide, Captain Jimmy Albright (I would later catch bonefish off the flat in front of Ted William's house at

Islamorada, a low-roofed, classic Keys home on a big piece of Atlantic-side waterfront, before he died). So of course I said yes to Rick. Not taking the offer would have been downright un-American. Damn right, I would go.

And there was something more personal involved. I'd fished with Rick for a week the previous year. I must have done something right. I had, through dedication and the acquiring of a skill, *earned* the honor. Otherwise he would have asked someone else from his growing legion of clients. I would be sure, of course, to tip Captain Rick Miller well at tournament's end, every penny that I could give. Ingratitude is, I believe, a suicidal quality, as it sometimes causes the homicide of the ungrateful. And I was definitely grateful that the Gold Cup was finally, after twenty-eight years, in its first year as a catch-and-release tournament. I could not imagine ever killing even one of these great fish, a species that can be as long-lived as a human being can, to satisfy a tournament's writ of *habeas corpus*, a delivery of the body as proof of life and capture, in death. It is abundantly clear they have it tough enough out there already.

If it were about the killing I would do it with a spear, anyway; thus outfitted, there have been many days whence I could easily kill enough to feed ten wives and one hundred children. This hunt has been done since man first walked at water's edge and it is simplicity defined. But we have complicated it a bit by insisting upon throwing flies at fish, particularly hardy marine fish. It is this very complication, this self-imposed difficulty that an angler must walk through that is the reason he does it. And because it is beautiful. Graceful, even; unless one is lobbing heavy flies with heavy rods to ridiculously huge fish that suddenly appear at the boat. It is also disarmingly effective under most angling situations, as fish, thank God, simply love to eat flies. How could someone kill the giver of such kind reciprocity? Contrary to the observationally popular belief of the chronically insecure, killing all that one catches does not increase one's penis size. Hunger is the one and only acceptable reason. I catch and consume plenty of speckled trout, *Cynoscion nebulosus* . They are delicate and delicious and, to the satisfaction of both the angling and scientific communities, nowhere near even threatened in status. Indeed, the trout, along with her cousin the redfish, ranks as the greatest success story *ever* in the history of wildlife and gamefish management; this, courtesy of angler Walter Fondren and the then-fledgling angler's group, the Gulf Coast Conservation Association of Houston. It was 1979 and by lobbying to give these popular but then disappearing species heralded gamefish status, in Texas waters at least, the trout and the redfish became immediately protected from commercial harvest. The fish's populations began a huge rebound which has not stopped to date. Other coastal states have followed Fondren's C.C.A. Texas model and had similar results.

Commercial harvest of tarpon, other than that for cat food in poor nations, should not be a concern, as she is, reputably, neither delicate in texture nor delicious in taste. No surprise, as frighteningly tough as she is. Loss of the coastal habitat she needs for the fostering of her babies in nursery areas is probably the greatest threat to the tarpon, as God stopped making warm, inviting waterfront property a long time ago. Yet thankfully, as with all game animals, those who hunt her and love her also fund the study of her and see to her continued health and prosperity as a species ("Tarpon Unlimited" is just such an organization, as is its sister group, "Bonefish Unlimited"). On a cold fiscal level the tarpon's life is, as all environmental worries are, a luxury of wealth looking for a cause.

The long-term view notwithstanding, simply hold a live tarpon's jaw in your hand. Unless one has no conscience, catching and releasing a tarpon is one of the most spiritual experiences given to us if we seek it to consummation. She huffs and puffs at the surface, breathing air in the fight if you let her, just like you probably are at the same moment. Feeling her struggle you know that both you and her have more than just a will to live. You have a spirit that transcends this, and you are now sharing it. Release her and you have an added satisfaction to the predator-prey relationship that simply must be experienced to be understood. You know more about what and where you and the tarpon are and, hopefully, nobody dies.

Anyone who has seen his own death, heart silent and interminable blackness surrounding him, finds it difficult to so much as hurt anything anymore, much less kill—especially a creature as noble and flat-out *cool* as our shark-tussling, air-breathing brother with fins, the tarpon.

* * * *

CHAPTER I

The Making of a Bonefisherman

There comes a moment in time for a man when one action, one irrevocable decision he makes, will define his character and his life. I have had two such moments, to date.

1985, my junior year:

"Roy, you're pretty messed up. Let me drive," I said to my friend, for the second time, as we left the clapboard pool hall on the outskirts of town, on our walk to the car for the drive back to our beloved Baylor University bubble. You've probably met me before: though far from innocent, I was the one of the group who watched his intake and maintained his snap—that sharp awareness of place and self driven by, at its core, preservation of life. Childhood illness and the recent, violent death of a high school friend to a drunk, illegal immigrant driver had immunized me against the youthful disease of imagined immortality that is replete on campuses everywhere. An added incentive to get home safely tonight was that Amy, my new girlfriend, was meeting me back at my apartment. We were just discovering each other and all things in such exploratory work are without a doubt better realized with a clear head. So I was being a good boy, ulterior motive notwithstanding.

Roy shook his head in a defiant "no way." Looking at him as he walked in front of me, I shook my own head. There was simply no talking to him. Pumped up at his massive shoulders with libation and testosterone, the two greatest contributors to that false sense of eternal life, he walked to the driver's side of the car, opened it, and like a big sack of potatoes he dropped his six-foot, five-inch frame into the driver's seat. I got in the back seat and strapped myself in with a noticeably insufficient lap belt.

Roy, too, had an ulterior motive that night: to thrash this fast little loaner car, a 1985 Chrysler Lebaron Turbo GTS he'd had for the week while his convertible was being serviced. But this, tonight, was a gravel road with sharp turns. "Roy, the turn," was the last thing I said, pointing. *Too fast, immortal one. You're going to get the bonus plan with this one.*. So we didn't make it around that first curve, a ninety degree banked hairpin that launched the little car up into the air. I felt the car and my stomach in a sickly unweighting at the apex, and then felt the rising downward velocity as we began to drop. It was all slow motion on the way down into the sunken cement culvert. I saw the impact looming. Looming.

Impact "on the nose" transformed the car into an amorphous, rounded mass of twisted steel, plastic and shattered glass that occupied about a third of its former space. The first and only sound I heard with the bone-snapping hit and then the rebound was the deep, peaceful snoring of Roy the driver and Brent, my roommate, in the front passenger seat. I looked at their profiles from my cubby hole in the back seat: like contented children in their unconscious slumber. As my head slowly filled with a buzzing pressure, I focused between my friends and saw two little pink posts imbedded solidly in the plastic center console. *Those are my front teeth—no shoulder straps in the back seat.* I was hyper-conscious, trapped inside a cracked capsule of shattered space, my head swelling with blood and claustrophobic terror. With the lower half of my broken femur pinned behind the buckled front passenger seat, I could not move. Time stopped. Panic filled inside my chest, adrenalin and fear. I felt as if I were constantly falling and that madness or death drifted just one scant moment ahead of me in time. I hovered there and listened to the unconscious snoring of Roy and Brent, and prayed that I quickly pass out, or die. Both dull and sharp pains throughout my head and body began to escalate in a throbbing pulse. I soon realized I had been deceived on a primal level for many years: passing out from pain is a myth parents must tell their children so all can sleep at night. I kept waiting for that "magic level" to be reached.

Then I heard a man hollering in the distance. There was a rural central Texas farmhouse I had noticed nearby, on our way out that evening. Mourning Dove had been everywhere, flying to roost. I felt a little hope. An eternity later, probably a real-time hour, I turned my head and looked into the eye of a man peering in at me.

His eyes roamed over my face and he said, "Oh my God." His jaw then hung slack. I made out his EMT uniform.

And I distinctly remember thinking, *You must be new or, please, please, look into another line of work.*

But he did get me out of that little space where I was losing both blood and sanity. And there by the ambulance at the crest of the culvert we'd flown down into was Amy. Someone must have put out a call. This was long before cellular telephones. She took one look at me on the stretcher and fell into histrionics. *Prognosis negative.* Everything I saw was flat and without depth. I did not realize it, but I had already lost one green eye, and the eye is an extension of the brain. So it could be argued that I did lose part of my mind that night, literally and figuratively. I finally lost consciousness, not from pain but from blood loss.

It was an E.R. surgeon wearing glasses talking at me that I awoke to. I was on a gurney in a busy white hub of hospital activity. Hillcrest Hospital, it was. Definitely the better of the two hospitals in Waco, Texas, at the time. The first thing I heard him say was that my father was coming to get me, which was both very professional and kind of him. I was instantly put more at ease. I asked about my friends. I didn't recognize my voice, or my own mouth, even. He gently pulled my hand away from my face. He told me that Roy and Brent had minor injuries and would be okay, but that the anesthesiologists were having difficulty putting them under for their procedures. They were fighting it, belligerently in fact. We went around about what his definition of "minor injuries" was for a while, and then he asked me, "in the strictest confidence," if I knew what my friends had taken on top of alcohol, that they be effectively put under. I remembered them taking and then offering me an Ecstasy tablet, and my refusing it. I simply did not enjoy the stuff. It was new and actually legal back then and I had tried it, and all it had done was scare the daylights out of me for several hours. It was far too serious a departure from reality for my tastes. I told the surgeon what they had taken, hoping its legal status created no legal problems. I was right.

The surgeon did not tell me what had happened to my body. He did tell me, however, that I had been easy to put under. Then he asked me why, on earth, had I not been the one driving. I told him I had tried. He shook his head and sighed in frustration, and I remember feeling as if everything had been my fault at that moment, that I should have tried harder, should have hit Roy over the head and taken the keys, perhaps. The surgeon looked at me and then smiled. He pat me on the hand and said he was only sorry it had happened, that it's impossible to make someone see reason when they are on that stuff, and that it was becoming frustrating for an emergency surgeon. I asked him what, exactly, had happened, to let me have a look in a mirror, and he raised his hands in a gesture of powerlessness over the lack of mirrors in a modern hospital, and told me not to worry, that no one would touch me at all anymore until my father arrived, unless it was absolutely necessary again, and he walked off. I was confused. No, my father is not a lawyer. He is a cardiovascular surgeon. I went out again.

I was transported to the Texas Medical Center. I woke up first to my father's voice, in Methodist Hospital, where an Irish surgeon with plump fingers had been trying to save my eye with his innovative, retinal re-associative surgeries. Dad stood in a whitecoat, talking to someone who obviously wasn't getting what he was saying. I felt safe, seeing him tear into someone.

Here I am again, where I was born. My father had been here that day, too, a Captain fresh out of the Army, in a neighboring operating theater, in a man's chest during the moment of my birth with his new boss and former cardiovascular surgery teacher, Dr. Michael DeBakey. I remembered that Dad had first thought working on Dr. DeBakey's team would be a less regimented life than that of the Army. "Boy, was I wrong on *that* one," he said with a smile, years later. So he had named me "Michael". After years with DeBakey, he teamed with Denton Cooley, and rounded out his best of the best exposure and education for his further pioneering of surgical techniques. The learning never ends in medicine, and Dad was there, in the middle of the creation of the new things that are today almost considered standard fare, as far as things that save one's life when a good heart or artery goes bad and absolute certain death looms can be considered "standard fare".

So Dad was here and I knew I was in the best of hands, because the best of hands only deal with the best of hands, once the "chaff" is eliminated. I went out again. I did that a lot over the next few weeks. The eye surgeon tried again and again with what was left of my retinal tissue to no avail. "It's the worst I've ever seen," he said. I didn't know it was possible to feel both proud and despondent at the same time. It is.

I was moved next door to St. Luke's, for the reconstructive facial bone work. Bones that had begun to set in my face and skull had to be pulled loose again, repositioned and then wired. New pains in old, reawakened places. It's best to be under general anaesthesia when pliers are used to torque the wires embedded in knitting facial bones. Ah, St. Luke's Episcopal:

I had been here just three months previously, when I'd walked the miles of white halls, looking at patients and nurses, and stood for still, precise hours in an operating theater with my father, as one allowable bonus of nepotism in my premedical studies. Dad kept the air temperature at sixty degrees for some procedures, to slow the flow of blood. This may have made him unpopular with some of his team, as surgery greens are scant insulation. But it was always about the patient, as it should be, with my father. The weak nurses and doctors were weeded out in many ways. One whose motive is personal comfort at all times, or the winning of fame and attention, should not go into the field of cardiovascular surgery, or any field of medicine for that matter.

Now, between surgeries, in demerol delusioned dreams, surgical instruments, shards of safety glass and steel shrapnel, all flew around me, at the center of a big white room, in a circular tornado. This was all about dreams and I remember not even having to consider it, that it was automatic: with no binocular vision or depth perception, any hands-on doctoring was simply out of the question. As a patient, the very thought of a one-eyed surgeon hanging over me and saying, "count back from a hundred," was more than disconcerting, it was nightmarish irresponsibility defined. But there was always psychiatry—as a patient. Better to think about that later. No. Medicine is gone. It is gone forever. And my other desire. What of that?

I had completed a qualified ground school with flight instrument training during my senior year in high school. Only then, after learning how to actually do it by the book and even do it in the dark, had I finally flown. It was a graduation gift. I remembered that after I had made some slow banked turns and he had shown me how to keep the plane level by keeping the earth's horizon in line with the dashboard, my instructor looked down in a log book of some sort in his lap at precisely the wrong moment that June day, when a low-wing twin-engine on its approach dropped down on top of our high-wing Cessna. It was looming right on top of us and there was no time to think. How serendipitous: I got the chance to really fly—it was that, or perish. I broke hard right and dropped the nose, and dove at full throttle, then quickly leveled off just in time to see the twin zip past our left, still on its path, its pilot apparently never having seen us at all.

"Wo," my instructor said, turning his head around to watch the twin on her way down, his hands locked to the dash in a death grip. He turned and looked to me in the left seat and smiled. "Didn't see that coming. Sorry." And then he told me something I will never forget. "Damn, I guess you can fly. That was pretty good." My mother, a pilot herself, was in the back seat, quiet as a church mouse.

After we landed he told me that I had avoided a classic, high-wing climbing, low-wing descending collision: blind zones for both pilots. "They happen a lot—if we're not paying attention and *someone's* not talking with the tower," he said, gesturing to a familiar-looking twin engine craft, freshly parked and unloading at a hangar. He went over the time and cost break down for training for my private license. I told him I wanted to fly jets, of course. Fast jets, and that I wouldn't necessarily mind it if people tried shooting at me.

I was given the choice of flying or college, and took college because of a scholarship that made it more affordable. But I would figure out a way to somehow do both, to slow down at some point, take a semester or two off and fly between undergraduate studies, or right after graduation but before medical school or military flight training on the taxpayers tab, for a big change.

In the electric hospital bed, I cracked a broken-toothed smile at the memory. Flying the F-15 Eagle, the bird of choice, was halted, so what was the point: fly Cessnas, and De Haviland Beavers and Otters in Alaska? Fact: that *would* be tame in comparison for a young man and, realistically again, one small fleck of dust, or a juicy Yukon mosquito, at precisely the wrong instant and that plane would crash and burn, too. I could not fly with a clear conscience knowing that I was simply and irrevocably physically compromised.

These dreams were now gone, pure folly. I know my mind was both practical and responsible in its assessments. While some would say continuing along these beloved career paths despite such setback would be courageous, I saw it instinctually for what it truly would have been: selfish. Other people could be hurt, or worse.

But such practical thinking was not conducive to the healing of my body and mind. I needed a good fantasy to keep me going. I was thankful for one very attractive "pet" nurse of one of my father's surgeon friends. She was auburn haired and always smiling, with a firm runner's body. She called me, "Kiddo." A lovely and also quite good nurse is of the highest value to a damaged young man. I remember thinking it should be required by law that, for all broken men who sense their lives are essentially over, they be tended by only the most qualified and beautiful nurses.

I had the best surgeons—not the cliché the medically ignorant extol, but the actual, most qualified surgeons who were the pioneers of the particular reconstructive procedures I needed. There was great comfort in that. But there was also the inescapable fact that the damage I had incurred did not leave these kind men much to work with. The best would be made of several bad medical situations; situations that would, however, remain bad. I was alive, and I would walk again. I would, eventually, be told that I should be thankful for that.

There are some things a man must be allowed to discover on his own. I felt no anger towards Roy; indeed, I felt guilty about my body failing me and being crushed. I didn't want to burden him with guilt. Anger would come later, much later. Anger at his being so intoxicated by a mind-altering substance that he would not listen to me, not listen to reason, right there in his ear, but instead would rather thrash a car under the pure delusion that we were immortal and that nothing bad could ever happen, that we would all just walk away from it and laugh because, well, that was *just damn well what he wanted to do and to hell with everything else.* Mission accomplished.

My thinking would be foggy for years to come from the blow to the head. But I already knew one thing for certain: one is overwhelmingly aware of the specific piece of earth one is on when maimed and dying. I had been on concrete, surrounded by it in a culvert, like a premeditated, concrete grave. I did not want to die on concrete.

I had just reached twenty-one years of age.

* * *

I went back to Baylor within a year. I could not possibly know whether I was ready or not, as I was the one with the head injury case making decisions with "damaged goods." I was not comfortable with my new face and new limp, and the new looks I got from the curious. Women I would have had no trouble with now looked the other way. I may have imagined half of it. I had the best surgeons, after all.

It was maybe that long period of panicked consciousness trapped in the tiny twisted back space of the car. The snoring. Just all the physical damage. Something might have snapped inside my head. *I will get as far away from concrete, steel, and people as is humanly possible, or I will die a very unhappy young man indeed.*

But I did not know where to start and I needed a push. So, that summer my dad took me trout fishing in the Colorado Rockies, not too far from the house my maternal grandfather built on top of Bear Mountain in the early fifties, where I'd later spent springs and summers as a child. It was a big, green and rocky piece of mountainscape in clear and dry blue sky on top of what would inevitably, like all nice country places removed from the far edge of town, become a suburb. Of Denver, in this particular case. It used to be Evergreen. Now it could be called "Some Green left", or just plain "Denver".

I always worked upstream so that I would be coming up from behind the trout, where I could often spot them looking upstream, unawares and unconcerned of what was behind them. I unconsciously sought a space alone, a distance away from David, my brother, and my father. My mind both lost and at peace in the aquatic world of the fish, I heeded to only one intention: fooling and catching each individual fish I spotted, or properly hitting each good-looking lie that I felt just *had* to hold a good brown, cutthroat or rainbow trout. I was, of course, partial to the calmer brown trout lies. They were more difficult to master.

My father had given me a great gift that summer indeed. The single-minded determination required to dupe certain "technical", or, as I called them, "problem", fish, left little room in a fractured head like mine for the sensation and interpretation of physical and psychological pain. This was much more to a broken young man than the standard, "solitude without loneliness," that fishing is to most, which His Honor Hugh Faulkus wrote of under his pseudonym, Robert Traver. No, fishing served as a big, temporary psychological eraser for everything in my troubled mind.

And one morning walking the shoreline below the dam of the Taylor River at a time of heavy water release, disappointed at finding few fish-able refuges for trout, I came upon a familiar looking man holding onto two perfectly spaced, perfectly hand-sized rocks in the middle of the torrent, his head held up high above the surface but with water nonetheless jetting up his chest in powerful rivulets into his nose, his legs trailing behind him on the surface of the current, chest waders slowly filling as pressurized water leaked past his lightly-cinched wading belt. His face, under the sheen of flowing water, was blue now, but he somehow kept clinging to the rocks. There were large boulders directly down current from him, boulders arranged like posts in a pinball machine. The pictures of sequence formed in my mind in an instant: waders filled, hands slacked, face underneath, drowned; then, bone-crushing impacts to a dead body for good measure. This was all very real and glib and there was no time now.

I walked into the water and, out of the corner of my one eye saw, not fifty feet away from me on my side of the river, a perfectly healthy looking man who was watching the drowning man. "Help me get him," I shouted to him as I hit the stronger current. I looked to the stranger again and he had not moved. I held out my hand to him, beckoning him to form a two man chain for if and when I slipped, but he would step no closer. I abandoned that idea and walked into the current alone, wondering what this drowning man had been thinking, going into the middle of the Taylor while the dam was dumping such a voluminous, anti-trout and anti-trout fisherman load of water and then I saw it: a calm pool with a nice feeder on the other side of the river. I also wondered what had happened to the perfectly healthy looking man to make him unable to overcome his fear and enter the current. I was in no shape to do this: though I had been back to walking again for a year now, the femur hadn't grown back straight and I waddled like a gimp duck, and I was down to 120 from 150 after having my jaw wired shut for two months so that my re-aligned and wired facial and jaw bones healed in proper alignment. But I somehow managed to hobble along stone to stone at blazing speed, like a gazelle, water to my waist like a sledgehammer, and was thankful that at least the ripping current had apparently pressured away most of the slimy algae. I reached the man, grasped him at the nape of the neck with my stronger, casting hand, the back of his fly vest and shirt a good handle, and like a cat grabs a kitten, I lifted his weight just as his big hands let go of the two rocks. He was now body surfing on the surface of the river with me as his guide and anchor. I walked him, surfing all the way, levitating really, into shore. He was unconscious and blue in the face, cyanotic, but breathing on his own. The one thing about Cardio-Pulmonary Resuscitation I remembered was that one does not perform it on someone who has a heartbeat and is breathing. I put him on his side to aid the draining of his lungs. He hacked with abandon.

Everything felt very crisp and vibrant now, on the shore, colors sharper, and I wondered how others in events where people were dying, because of their mental detachment and physical in-actions, their decision or, indeed, their simple physical reaction to do nothing, must not believe that they even have a horse in this race called life to begin with.

I felt irrefutable proof of God for a moment there, on the bank of the Taylor: I was not in the physical world, walking to the drowning man in the river; I was above it. All impeding thought was simply overridden. Not any thing of this earth could have stopped me from saving him. A man could have had my head squared in a rifle scope's reticle, pulled the trigger and that bullet would have been denied entry, been obliterated into a powder of lead dust, "Pooof," as I was above the physical realm.

That drowning man in the Taylor River was my father. When he came to on the river bank, he said, "It's not true what they say, that you see your life flashing before you...just see blackness." Dad thanked the man who had stood at the edge of the river's current. Yes, he had walked over after I had my father safely ashore. The man said, "Oh, just a fisherman helping a fisherman," and bathed in full credit looking quite the humble man. The wind left my chest and I was completely disarmed. I felt a deep resignation and indefinable loss wash through me. I knew, of course, what had really humbled him: his insurmountable fear. Such a repugnant force is as real as earth, fire, blood and water in some people, I had just shockingly learned. This man shook my father's hand and said his name was Bill, Bill Bell.

After I loaded my father into our truck, Bill walked up to me, out of earshot of my father, and bowed his head meekly and said, "you know you saved his life, son, don't you?"

"Yes," I said, and turned away from him. I got into the truck and drove away.

Seeing my father in the river, my only thought was to keep a man from drowning. There was no time to contemplate how life would be without him. I knew he had been suffering horribly: the panic that accompanies drowning, one's very soul desperately, hopelessly fighting against a rushing, thundering, inescapable "this is it" departure, is as devastatingly terrifying as the fiery burning of water in one's lungs. Yes, I almost drowned, too, in the Medina River on some old family land.

And so I learned that acts of personal risk are not acts that, aw, shucks, anyone else would do under the circumstances—Mister Anyone Else had been standing right next to me at the time, and he did nothing. Bill must have felt he had no personal stake, no real thing to lose. Sure, he had no courage to begin with so there was no losing of what he never possessed, but there is *always* something to lose. I thank God for making me, and many others, different from Bill.

Driving back home I saw a sign along the bank that read, "Dangerous current: do not wade during heavy dam release".

"No shit," I said to myself, and pointed to the sign for my father to read. He laughed as much as a light blue, water-logged man who had just lost a thousand dollar fly rod outfit could laugh, and I knew he would be all right after a hot bath and a big scotch. We drove in silence. I know he felt ashamed of the frailty of his own life, strong as he was—and believe me, no one on earth has stronger hands than a thoracic surgeon. He needn't have felt this, and I wanted to wash it away from him, as I already knew the fragile nature of every life. I had been recently dead, myself, after all.

"Dad, that man didn't do a damn thing back there," I finally said.

I did not know whether he believed me or not; he was, after all, unconscious at the time, which is a state of being that pretty much defies all criticism. Besides, I knew I would look, physically, a lot, lot worse if it had not been for him, and his surgeon buddies.

So indeed, blood is thicker than water, and I do not trust strangers I meet on rivers in any matters of importance.

I became confused and uncomfortable about everything in this world but fish. I would seek their company in abandonment of all others.

* * *

CHAPTER II

GEORGE

The Caye Bokel bonefish were surfing on that blustery November morning. The previous afternoon they had fed with unusual abandon on the island's reef flat, where George and I had teamed to successfully interrupt the dining of many individuals with my fly rod. I had lost count; George, being the typical guide in at least his observance of numbers and size of fish, had not: fifteen, three to five pound bonefish hooked, played and released in the space of two or three hours. One of the first we released had unfortunately been taken by a loitering, opportunistic barracuda before we even knew he was on the scene. George, shouting in broken Creole and English, had run after him with arms flailing and chased him off. Nevertheless, we kept our eyes up and held the next bones in the water a little longer after the episode of double-predation.

With nine days of decidedly more relaxed angling behind us, such heightened food chain activity had tweaked our curiosity. And that night, our answer had arrived in the form of a massive wind shift out of the north. The air temperature dropped to fifty-eight degrees, and hung there for a few hours. It was short-lived, and had climbed back up above seventy degrees—the minimum preferred *water* temperature of bonefish—soon after sunup.

And now, under a bluebird, high-pressure sky and blazing sun, an out of place arid wind still howled out of the north as George Morales and I stood near the lagoon-side top of the purple and green, turtle grass carpeted coral reef, and watched the bonefish as they surfed: facing into the current of an incoming tide that fought against the Northern, each fish in the big school would rise up nose-first above the water's surface to meet with every gently breaking, wind-torn wave where, at its little crest, the fish would briefly cut sideways to ride the roller for a half-second before submerging and heading back out over the reef top. The Marlboros I had brought from the States that we had been smoking long gone, George and I shared a Belizean Independence cigarette, and watched.

"They must be happy," I theorized aloud. "Or maybe they're just worried about scraping their fat bellies on the coral. Hmmm…"

"They do that sometimes with a big weather change, Jim," George said.

I looked to him, and he was visibly pleased to see that the fish were behaving according to his winter model *in extremus* . George had twenty years of guiding the islands of this Belizean archipelago under his belt, whereas I had a mere nine days of fishing here as a client. I was in a constant state of wonder. After what had happened to my body, what it had done to my mind, my normal mental state was one of physical uncertainty and insecurity, with brief moments of terror. Feeling safe with George, I had been able to give myself to wonder.

"They take, George?" I asked, as I tore the filter butt from the burned cigarette paper and put it into my carry-along ash tray, a Ziploc quart bag. George shook his head ever so slightly and smiled at my gesture, thinking I didn't see him doing it again. I'm an environmental smoker. The extra hydrocarbons and carbon dioxide I exhale provide the green plants of Kingdom Plantae with much needed fuel for photosynthesis. I learned this fact in Premedical Biology. I'm not sure what the trace cyanide does, however. Maybe, "what doesn't kill you, makes you stronger," applies to plants. Mostly I've just never littered, as one has simply either been given a respect for the world and what is not his or he has not, and the idea of a bonefish swimming up to and curiously sniffing a floating cigarette butt makes me sick. It damned sure won't be mine.

"Yeah, mon," he answered. "If you put it to them right, they eat your fly."

Fifty to seventy feet away, and with a ripping tail wind, it should have been an easy shot; but I could *not* get the fly to them. I did not know it but my back cast, without focus of power on the stop, was opening up in the bracing wind behind me and as a result I was bringing slack noodles of fly line and leader forward. I knew nothing of the Belgian cast, a cast with a tight, swing-around back cast that works wonders with a tail wind. So, cast after futile cast, my presentations were collapsing short, or, even worse, dumping upon the bonefish like bowls of overcooked spaghetti thrown into the wind. It degraded from there, too: the fish would not spook away, as any normal bonefish would do. Oh, no, they hung around the reef top, surfing away, waving their silver sides and tails at me. Ten minutes of failure passed. Frustration finally peaked and a breaker switch in my damaged head tripped.

"Aaarrrrghhhh!" I snapped, blowing the promising day in bad form. "George, take this rod away from me or I'll crack it in half."

I turned to hand the rod to my guide, and saw that his eyes were looking down, staring into the water. "Jimmy, Jimmy," he said, shaking his head.

"Oh, hell. They got to me, George," I said. "Let's have a Beliken. I need to chill out."

George's eyes immediately came up, with a smile. "I think that's a good call," he said. He knew he would get to rest on the skiff for an hour and drink a beer while his client probably had two. I had found that the alcohol, while it didn't actually do much to reduce pain, did, however, do an excellent job of taking my mind off it.

"You were doing so well, yesterday," George said.

"It crept up on me, George," I said. We gently walked down inside the reef top onto the sand and sea grass flat of Caye Bokel, where we had gotten into the numbers just a short day before. I made a point of keeping the fly rod in my hand, squeezing the Portuguese cork, as we slowly waded back to the skiff, a half mile further down the reef top. Although George had lost three fingers from his right hand in a lumberyard accident as a boy, it was not as if I would be burdening him with the rod: he was used to carrying even the redundant gear of obsessive-compulsive clients. I wanted to hold onto it. Walking over the sea grass, I listened to the light crunching noise our feet made through the water as we collapsed the little tubes of dead coral particles that are made by the many intertidal zone animals, worms, shrimp, and other creatures, as they dig underneath and deposit the stuff above them, and wondered how long it takes the little animals to rebuild the entrances to their little lairs. I was hit with a flash of anger at any and all destruction. I turned around to watch the last bonefish in the school as they surfed and swam out over the reef top. "I'll be back. I swear it and I'll catch you," I said, pointing the rod at them for emphasis. I made a quiet commitment to find a mentor and get a more formal, hands-on casting education.

George gave me a concerned sideways glance. *This is a strange one*, he must have thought to himself. He spoke of a secret spot for snook on the western, lee side of the archipelago. He kept it to himself that fishing for them, relaxed in the skiff, would allow me to rest more. George was good at reading a client's limitations, even the troubled ones, and because of this there was rarely any need he felt to hold their hands and supplicate to them. It was keystone in George's relaxed and successful *Angler management*.

He had begun a yearly odyssey with me, one during which he would witness a search for wildness that had started healthily as it grew relentlessly and insidiously into focused, single-minded obsession. This was, after all, in his job description, and it was possibly the most compelling reason he had become a guide in the first place: *for the ride*. Why else might a man spend day after day on a skiff and almost never get to fish himself for a few hard-earned American dollars? Well, every now and then he gets to see a grown man absolutely fold up in front of him, lose it and practically go back to the womb psychologically. So he gets to see this and then, if his angler is dedicated, he gets to see him work through it and overcome the weaknesses. Maybe then even, they actually grow into a *team*. Having to go through the rough spots is just plain ugly though, waiting through it until it can be looked at with the gift of hindsight as the necessity it was. Maybe after that they can laugh, and appreciate the pain—if there is some victory in the end and nobody gets seriously hurt. Nevertheless, with me at his side, George's forecast must have been *bumpy as Hell*.

I absolutely loved working as a team. And I needed my guide's eyes.

* * *

CHAPTER III

CHUCK

It is both written and spoken mantra that the angler should learn everything on the lawn with the fly rod before he ever gets to the fishing grounds, where his capability and his very manhood will be held in judgment by fish and fishing guides, let alone by himself. But what better motivation is there than occasional humiliation to keep one from repeating such embarrassing historical events? Looking back on my angling education, I would not have altered its course in almost any way whatsoever, even if I had had the impossible option of a crystal ball and a way to manipulate away those golden moments that most anglers prefer to dismiss or just flat-out deny.

* * *

"Bonefish, huh," Chuck said. "I'm sure they're tough but there's a redfish right in front of you and if you don't thread the needle and put it right in front of her nose in that thick grass you won't have a chance. She'll never see dinner if you don't deliver. So get His Royal Highness Sir Bonefish out of your mind for now, Jimbo, and focus."

I shot a thirty or forty foot cast out, locked down on the fly line, and snapped Chuck's fat bend back fly right in front of the redfish in question, let it sink through the Texas turtle grass, twitched the fly as if it were afflicted with Parkinson's, and watched the fish charge it like a bull and eat it. Accuracy is the most important piece of equipment, anywhere, any target species, but this seems to be especially true with redfish. Captain Chuck Scates reinforced this fact to me, almost as much as the fish themselves (my personal observations lead me to conclude that denser marine vegetation and water that is often more turbid than typical bonefishing waters necessitate putting the fly closer to redfish than bonefish; that a redfish could see just fine if he weren't rooting up to his gills in grass and marl all the time).

And Chuck did not need to hear about bonefish while he was putting me on redfish after feeding redfish in six inches of clear, sea grass bottomed Laguna Madre water. No, that was the disrespectful, blaspheming talk of a head-injury case still in the process of knitting his mind back together. I had hurt his pride by extolling the supremacy of the bonefish while on his water.

But fish and guides tend to be forgiving. And a healing moment was holding that beautiful Texas Redfish, taking in the spots—the ocelli—just forward of her almost luminescent, neon blue-tipped tail, feeling her ironclad bulk—a redfish is an incredibly muscular, substantial fish with knife-dulling scales.

Holding the fish, I remembered that George had said I was dropping my back-cast from time to time, particularly when I was tired. I had paid little attention and so, earlier on this day, having no doubt observed the same thing, Chuck had simply stepped down from his poling platform, walked up to me on the bow, where I was encased inside his custom netted casting platform, and asked me to give him my casting hand. I had obliged, and he'd promptly strapped a leather bondage device, a Simms Wrist-Lock, onto my wrist. I immediately knew what it meant: my casting sucked. I was crushed, absolutely devastated. Fly fishing had already sneaked up on me and become the most important thing in my life. It was almost my very identity, which was now having a crisis.

"Slow down," Chuck said. "Your loop does everything that your wrist does, Jim. I think you're opening up your wrist on the back cast when you're tired," he pantomimed, "which opens up the fly line loop behind you, and as a result you're bringing complete slack forward on your forecast and trying to present trash to the fish."

Point taken. I was embarrassed and humbled; but it worked. I do not believe that I have ever, not once, opened up my back cast anywhere near Chuck since that day. I know that somewhere, close at hand, lurks that Hannibal Lector leather device of humiliation. Good guides are direct.

With my thumb opening her rubbery mouth, I ran the redfish forward and then gently backward in the water until she shivered and then kicked herself free. I had found happiness, a reason to live in angling. All involved elements feel perfect together, as if they were made explicitly for each other—this water for this fish, this tide for this fish, this sea grass for hiding this type of shrimp, these flies to imitate this kind of shrimp for this fish, this fly line for this rod, this rod for this angler. Each of these ingredients all come together to make the absolute, best game in the world, and I have found it. This is, I know in my heart, healthy obsession and I hope every human finds what it is that makes this same thing happen inside him.

Nevertheless, I sought out the chief guru of fly casting. Enough of humiliations.

CHAPTER IV

MEL

"You should keep it all in here, like this—especially with that shoulder of yours, Jim," Mel Krieger said, taking my rod and hand into his. I felt his smooth acceleration, and then a heart-beat stop of the rod on both the forward and back casts. The physics of casting a fly rod immediately registered to me in a light bulb moment.

He stepped back to watch me cast.

"A good cast," he said. "But not a great cast, Jim."

Startled, I turned to look at him, but he was already walking away, over to the next student, his back square to me.

I had just been challenged. Mel is not subtle. And he is very effective. "Practice and you'll get it—there is no substitute," Mel's very character exuded. He talked of muscle memory and lower brain stuff. "Keep that cerebrum out of it—you'll fail if you think about it too much," was the gist.

So I essentially took a semester off from Baylor, and each and every day for two months I went to the nearby Brazos River and practiced casting, stopping only at the point when self-defeating, defect saturation was at hand each day.

"I'll show you a great cast, Mel," I muttered to myself, those first few frustrating days. But with each successive day at casting time, I found I was pulling my Sage rods from their socks with increased anticipation for the wonderful feeling of rod loading and unloading, and the line and fly actually going where I commanded them. Single-mindedness and a fragile, slighted ego propelled me forward and frustration was replaced with skill. With my new casting shoulder, one reconstructed by an apparent genius named Malcolm Granberry, I was actually becoming a jock. For effort I received result. But, as I had learned directly from Mel and the bonefish and the redfish, I needed constant challenge to keep me in a hungry, learning mode, and to keep from falling into self-doubt.

In saltwater fly fishing I had willingly chosen an unequaled teacher of humility: there are fish that can and do literally beat up an angler, fish that snub the most perfect presentation of the perfect fly, and elemental conditions of weather, sea and wind that can combine to defy the most skilled caster.

And with this intentionally difficult search for life at its most elemental, there were times I felt truly happy again, when anger and sadness vanished in moments of bliss.

✻ ✻ ✻

CHAPTER V

GEORGE, and Unfinished Business

"Oh, I cannot believe this!" George wailed from the bench at the back of the skiff (there was no high-dollar aluminum platform). He pushed us down the flat with his hand-carved mangrove push pole, hitting each stroke hard for emphasis . "The Golden Bonefish, Jimmy! You had him! That would be a free trip back to the lodge for you, and a feather in my cap with the other guides, too. " He shook his head and stared into the water. "God, help us," he said.

"My bad, George. Sorry," I said. It was a conspiracy of laziness and brain damage that had lost the Golden Bone, and I truly felt horrible about it, for him and myself.

I had just lost an incredibly rare fish: There is a rare genetic mutation of _Albula vulpes_ that lacks the genes to produce normal pigment, and is, in effect, an albino bonefish. I've never heard of them existing anywhere else in the world except for this Turneffe Island Archipelago population of bonefish. Isolation of such individuals within a population would make the recessive mutation more likely to pop up, in fact (I learned such useful knowledge in my pre-med. Genetics studies). I had seen three of them, or the same fish three times, hunting different flats on the southern quarter of the archipelago during my twenty days here, up to that time (I'd always stay past the regular angling week, and leave with the supply boat for four extra days of fishing). The guides still debate over how many there are at any given moment. The mutants are typically bigger than average bonefish, and each time I've seen them, they've either been located in the middle of a school, or at the very lead of it when hunting; such location providing either a buffer of body protection, or more early notice of a predator, re-spectively. They must know they stand out like sore thumbs, or surely they would not survive long enough to get above three or four pounds.

Minutes ago, at the beginning of the flood tide, I had cast a pink, #8 Mini-puff to a golden bonefish that we'd spotted at the head of a small school milling in a depression named "Joe's Hole", inside the reef flat of big Caye Bokel, and he'd taken it aggressively. I'd set the hook and he'd proceeded to run his first hundred-yard dash when my knot, an improved clinch, "pig-tailed"—the wraps I'd put into it were simply too few and they'd slipped loose under strain, coming off the hook and leaving a ghostly reminder of my error on my tippet in the form of a series of curly-cues. The pigtail is irrefutable proof. The golden bonefish had then swum right past the skiff, still at the head of his school, and we could plainly see the pink fly sticking out of the corner of his mouth. He looked to be around five or six pounds. He was otherworldly, ethereal to my eye. I swear that I could see his brain through his pigment-free head. I found comedy in the conspiracy of manifested genetic fish error and human error: If ever there were a gay-looking bonefish, this pale golden mutant with that splash of pink in his jaw—the visually loud fly a symbol of his coming out of the closet and proudly proclaiming his uniqueness, perhaps—as he swam over the forest of green turtle grass in that one little window of life-altering time, was it. He was the gay king, and I was the big loser.

In the quiet time of reflection on my ineptitude and the absorption of loss, I looked to George. He was noticeably stunned. I fetched him a bottle of Beliken from the bottom of our lunch cooler. "Why's it called 'Beliken' again, George?" I asked him, though I knew the answer. I liked to hear him say it.

"Because, 'pelican, pelican: his beak can hold more than his belly-can,'" he smiled, tipping back the beer. We laughed for a moment.

"George, this game is so intense," I said. "How do you do it, day in and day out—especially after your anglers do stupid things like I just did?"

"Jimmy," he said. He shook his head and exhaled a long breath. "First, I know what I am. I'm a black man who works to find fish for other men, white men mostly, but I get the satisfaction of giving them the best shot I can—like to the Golden Bone there. It means more than if I cast to them myself. I guess that makes me a freak. But I learn a lot about these men when it's tough, under pressure, and myself. It is gold in my hand. It is a bigger thing than color."

"A diver at the lodge asked about it and I tried to explain it to him. He said it was just flat-out racism and animal abuse: white angler, black guide poling the boat around all day, abusing defenseless fish."

"Hah," he laughed. "That's just because black Caribes live here, so of course they guide here. I fish with white guides from America all the time, and they tip good, too. I got a brand new fly rod from your river guide in Montana, matter of fact, and *that's* something impossible to get here."

"They all work hard, so they know."

"Shoot, diver has black deck hands on the dive boat, and I know he doesn't tip them like anglers tip their guides. He doesn't fish. He can't know."

"Well, at least he's curious," I said, and then made a show of inspecting my fingernails. "And, I heard he booked a half-day's fishing with Joe tomorrow."

George rolled his head back and laughed. "Bet he never dives again," he said.

I looked into the impossibly clear Caribbean water at the turtle grass in the shallow basin we floated on, at the tiny flashing flecks of neon light that suspended in the water, plankton, flitting and turning about the green blades with the incoming tide, and out of the corner of my eye I saw the school of bonefish, regrouped now after the ruckus of hooking and losing their mutant king. They swung around the basin's edge, reached out higher with the rising water, and quickly angled up and onto the reef flat proper. They began to feed, exposing their tails in the shallower water of the flat on the flood.

I gave George my fly rod. After losing the golden bone, I had properly tied on a #8 metallic green Nasty Charlie, a hot fly that George promptly bit the bead-chain eyes off of so that they would not snag on the grass blades, sponges, sea fans, or other uprisings on the flat. Thus altered it became a "Blind Charlie", and it was excellent for combat fishing in inches of obstruction-filled water. Though a small fly, an elephant will indeed eat a peanut.

George got out of the skiff and waded towards the bonefish, which were now absorbed in "setting up" their feeding pattern. Right handed, he cast with the thumb and index finger of his unique hand—it is the opposable thumb that makes this possible, he says. I watched as the fly touched down with a tiny "plip" of water. The bones did not spook. Squatting low to the water as the fish approached him, he began to strip the line and the fly. He hooked one and raised the rod up high to protect the leader from the coral, and as the fish screamed off in a long run, a white raised rooster tail of water climbed into the air after the departing fly line and created the sound of ripping Velcro in the air. George wailed in boyish happiness. I smiled. It wasn't the golden bonefish—he would be careful about what he ate for a while yet—but it was a nice bonefish of around five pounds. I had denied us gold but had at least tendered silver to my guide and friend. This was the most meaningful bonefish of that trip to me.

During that late December, 1990 night, as in the previous year, an arctic front reached down through the Central Flyway and pushed through Belize. The following morning with clear skies, rising temperatures and an incoming tide, George and I found ourselves with the Caye Bokel surfing bonefish again. This time, I had the Belgian cast in my arsenal, and used it without even having to think about it. I bagged my surfing bonefish while George, at my side, announced my victory over the great evil of mediocrity. It was a banner day.

* * *

That night, George invited me over and we celebrated Boxing Day at the guides' quarters after the main lodge had locked up for the night. We tied flies that got progressively uglier and more desperate-looking with time and rum. We ran out of the rum and, coincidentally, there was a "break in" at the main lodge's liquor cabinet. In the morning the scuba divers, as they walked down the pier to their dive boat, were greeted by the sight of one of the native revelers, passed out at the threshold of the Lodge's Bertram shuttle boat, the *Grand Slam*, next to a pool of his own vomit and his hastily packed luggage. As I walked down the pier to George's skiff, I slowed to look at the presently prone and unconscious young man, surrounded by a crowd of vacationing scuba divers, and remembered during the party he had voiced his intent to avenge a wrong done him by someone back on the mainland, and his basic dissatisfaction with life out here in the keys. I'd said to him, "Then why don't you get back to the mainland. The supply boat runs on Wednesdays—that's when I leave, too." Apparently he could not wait, as this was a Monday. Any soul desperate enough could have fired up one of the lodge's many boats. This man had almost made it to freedom, and certain death.

I looked down the pier and saw George sitting in the idling skiff, beckoning me to hurry with his crippled hand, his other on the throttle. He was laughing, absolutely beaming like the Cheshire cat, and shaking his head from side to side. I paced quickly on down to him, hopped in the skiff, and while I was stowing my four fly rods George hit the throttle and we were off, no time for pleasantries.

We both heard someone calling over the outboard, over our shoulders, "Hey, you! Wait! Stop!"

George and I, we didn't turn around. We got the hell out of there. Went fishing.

I had become an instigator, a trouble-maker.

* * *

The act of casting a fly rod had, as with most any athletic skill, begun its transition through the psychological "wall of failure". It was no longer necessary that I first make a big analysis and a plan of attack before a cast, often through a struggle of conscious effort, and then follow this by an appropriate or, just as likely, inappropriate cast for the given conditions; no, it was becoming an act of instinct and reaction, free of premeditation and self-doubt. This is the critical point in an angler's career where he will either stop development and be contented to live in mediocrity, or he will step his game up and walk through the wall of self-imposed limitation to a freedom of release that lies on the other side of himself.

There are the technical casters, those who have the physics of the cast ingrained in their muscle memory and are pretty to watch—in a vacuum, that is; for confronted with a brisk wind for the first time these controlled-environment boys will fold up. I was here once, though I did not feel pretty even when I was told that I was by my mentors. Another interesting type of caster is the fishing-practical caster, who adapts with conditions and fishes fairly effectively in the salt water realm. These tenacious pilgrims have limits, however, such as distance and speed of delivery to the target; both of which are vital in saltwater angling. They are busy in their lives off the water and typically cannot dedicate themselves to find the time for improvement. And then there is the rare combination of the two: the predators. These anglers are the real weapons. At this time, in 1991, I was a technical caster stubbornly banging away at the wall, and already reaping rewards: I was making some difficult shots and bagging fish. But I was obsessed by shots I missed, the ones I could not make specifically because of the way the wind blew in any given scenario. This immediately put me into indecision and created a mental block, a hesitation that is deadly in this game of speed. But I was in self-competition, striving to better my casting, which is the proper, pure motive for any pursuit. A saving grace of perpetuity is that I always come back to this; it is one reason I still fish and continue to get something out of it, even when I fail. But at this time a certain character type approached and threw me off kilter: the competitive fishermen, the "sport".

The "little wager on the side" types always made their approach on the dock at the end of the day, or in the dining room with an audience if they were especially bold. I must not have looked very intimidating, hobbling along the dock with my fly rods and grinning happily like a half-wit: I was still a fairly naïve young man in my twenties, after all. But in my youth, damaged though I may have been, the power of testosterone was nonetheless indomitable and I was taken aback by these decades-older, yet nonetheless still cocky types who brought their competitive world out here, onto the flats, and put angling on a plane with money and one-up-manship. I never refused a challenge. Hey, these strangers *challenged* me and my guide. Each time, I felt I had been approached by something dirty and corrupt. Perhaps they would learn that gambling on bonefish was a bad idea in principle after they lost enough times. I got them at the door with terms: these were catch-and-release, word of honor bets with our guides as witnesses, and the loser would pick up the winner's bar tab for the day, or the week. I soon wanted to beat them into submission for having cheapened the very thing I lived for.

So in our third year together, George and I had become "Team Gimp", what with George's two-fingered hand, my cyclopean head and other irreparables. And we would remain *undefeated* Team Gimp. But I was not *that* good. I just wanted to beat them more than they wanted to beat me. No challenger could stand losing for more than two days before "shutting the game down". Apparently my psychology was working: losing made them go away. And it also served to intimidate into silence most other potential comers who might be lurking in that week's batch of anglers for the rest of their stay. George and I could fish in peace once again. Until the next week's batch arrived.

In the brief reign of Team Gimp, I began to look at each bonefish as a notch on my rod, a fish against my rival's fish, a number to defeat corruption, and not a real fish, a creature of God. I caught myself in time. The coup de grace occurred one very slow, bad weather day when a sixty-something challenger brought his one, dying bonefish back to the dock. He had the small fish tied to a heavy leader behind the skiff, and claimed he merely wanted to photograph it and show it to the scuba divers—but they saw schools of bones off the reef on their dives, I knew. The truth was he did not trust us and wanted to see the bodies, despite his guide's uncomfortable and humble protest that he could trust the word of my guide. The wind left my chest as I saw—indeed, I could almost *smell* this wonderful gift of a way of life decomposing underneath my very nose. I was disgusted with him and myself. He eventually took his guide's, George's, and my word of our own paltry, five bonefish day, and we took his drinks with impunity. Everyone felt insulted. Something pure and beautiful had been deflowered.

Team Gimp talked it over that night and that was the end of it for us with gambling on bonefish. What was next? Dynamite angling? Fishing with *Eau de Crab* Spray ? Shutting it down was all for good; and perhaps we would be a more effective team without drinking all of those free drinks, come to think of it. A couple of those days we had gloated a bit heavily, too, victory over the corrupt and all. I hated it. Their drinks were like poison to my soul.

At the end of each challenge I gave the vanquished a few of my smaller, subtler and more effective patterns, out of pity and penance. Bonefishing must remain uncorrupted. It is a spiritual experience with spiritual creatures. It is a man alone on a shallow, saltwater flat under the sun with a modified form of one of the two most ancient and most effective angling tools ever created: the hand line, with a long lever to deliver to a spooky fish a tuft of bird feathers and hair on a hook. When someone gets haughty-taughty about fly fishing being an elite sport, I remember that, at heart, it is just glorified hand-lining. And as such it is the purest angling method. It is purer than any rod outfitted with a mechanical winch, a product of modern technology. Fly fishing is also the most difficult and challenging method, which is, of course, why I and many others choose it and forsake all others. It simply feels *right*.

The other ancient method, of course, is the spear. If I were still a betting man I'd put my money on the bonefish, every time, against a spear-chucking "angler". While a grisly prospect, we needn't fear: such a method isn't a true challenge because the fish has no say in the matter, which is an absolutely indispensable part of a precious game. The animal must oblige us willingly and, at the highest evolution of the game, he does this by honoring our own, hand-tied flies. Now that's *doing* something. That's *earning it.*

CHAPTER VI

EDDIE

The permit hunts with his nose, and a fly doesn't smell right. You must provoke him to strike. But two, three of them together, and they compete for the fly—if it suits them at the time.

——-Eddie Hyde, thirty-five year flats guide, Turneffe Archipelago, Belize, C.A., 1989.

It was my second trip to Turneffe, in 1990, during which I would first meet a species of fish that would forever change my life. It was the second Saturday when George had to run to Belize City on the supply boat to see his wife for a family concern, and I would fish with Eddie for the next four days. Eddie was a very quiet man until something happened between us that broke the ice. We went far north on a couple of those days, past Nelson's Caye, close to the agreed-upon, self-imposed proprietary fishing boundary established for neighborly relations between the two lodges of the archipelago, Turneffe Island Lodge in the extreme south, and Turneffe Flats to the far northeast. We may have been in a gray area on a couple of occasions, as I actually saw a Turneffe Flats Lodge boat for the first time, ever. We all waved, but we knew someone had maybe crossed a line somewhere.

There was an old Caribe on Nelson's Caye named Mister Banner who had two young daughters that occasionally visited him from Belize City, and also several pigs that ran wild on the island. The hogs would sometimes root around right at the shoreline, with bonefish tailing a few yards away. Mister Banner sold coconut oil and ham for a living, I was told, which made perfect sense. The first time I saw him he was standing on his dock when Eddie cut inside the reef to fish the flat in sight of his clapboard shanty, where a school could almost always be counted on with an incoming tide, and where a golden bonefish was sometimes spotted. We waved to him at our trespass. The tide was up high and Eddie poled the skiff right up to the white coral sand beach and paralleled it slowly, cutting in and around the few individual mangrove shoots. We spotted a bonefish at the same time, a big single over the white coral sand right at the beach, hunting so shallow his dorsal fin and half his back were in the air. So oriented, he was an "eyes forward", technical fish. He was slowly working his way towards us, turning this way and that in and around the mangrove shoots, actively feeding. Sometimes things just work and I dropped a decidedly small fly with a perfect "plip" that sent a tiny drop of water into the air, about six feet in front of where this fish was casually headed. I let it sink to bottom. When a fish just doesn't have a clue that there's something devious going on and he's a mere thirty feet away in such clear water, he will reveal his true nature when he sees a prey item, or a good fake. Once he approached it within a foot or so, I stripped the fly in a tiny one inch hop, picking it up off the bottom, and this now obviously large bachelor bonefish's fins shot up and out in excitement and he uncontrollably threw himself onto the fly, inhaling it quickly, before it could get away. I felt the resistance, struck him, and he reacted with a run towards the open flat and the reef, a half mile away.

Eddie exhaled in obvious relief and said, "You not hook him, they would have laughed at you, Jimmy." I looked to him briefly, push pole in hand as he turned the skiff towards the fish's exodus run, and saw him nod his head towards Mr. Banner. His daughters had come out on his dock to watch with him. They had been watching the entire stalk, some hundred yards away.

"How'd they know, that far away?" I asked.

"They see people fish here all the time. They know. Give my anglers a hard time they blow it," he smiled. "Scared to come over here sometimes. They can make it a pretty tough week, they laugh at my angler."

"Well, thank God for this fish then, Eddie. Thank God indeed. His daughter's nice to look at?"

Eddie laughed. He was talkative from then on. That bonefish went seven pounds.

And from then on, whenever we would run this far north, I made a point of stopping at Mr. Banner's rickety dock to give him Marlboro cigarettes and a cold Beliken.

Further inside the reef's lagoon near Nelson's, Eddie knew of a mile-long ridge, a continuous stair step a foot or two tall, that traversed a big sea grass flat that had a few small mangrove hummocks riding along the step. With a moving tide, water either tumbled over this ridge, or eddied as it rose up above it, either of which confused and tossed bait around, particularly crabs—the permit's seductress and delicacy. I had seen these elegant fish before, with George, but only as they were fleeing whatever scene we happened to be on at the time. They swam around drop offs and the deeper edges of the flats, and sometimes we would briefly see them as they suspended over huge purple coral heads at the reef's extreme southern edge, at the end of the inside reef flat of big Caye Bokel, where the coral wall suddenly ended and plunged to the deep blue depths of the Western Caribbean. Permit looked like tall, silver, half-sized ironing boards with huge eyes and a starkly black tail shaped exactly like a sideways "Y" when they swam. The tail never stopped beating back and forth, back and forth, like a metronome. I had never seen these fish sit still. They were phantoms of movement, permit. I was told by my guides that, at the time, there were *maybe* close to three hundred people in the world who had ever caught one on a fly.

Today, the tide was tumbling over the step along the sea grass flat and we'd see the black sickle tail thrashing about in the air right at its edge, and know we'd have about as good a shot at a permit any man can ask for. Obsessed with consuming crabs at the mercy of the tide, the permit behaved with utter depravity and gluttony. They'd surely be more likely to eat a fake at this feeding trough. Watching them in such a desperate state eroded their phantom, mythical status in my eye, and, temporarily, at least, put them in perspective: they were hungry fish on the feed at the dining table, like southern boys engrossed with a bucket of fried chicken. They would be much more likely not to take the time to smell every offering before them in their haste, much more likely to eat a fake, we hoped.

I lost three enormous permit in the space of two hours. Angler failure was the killer with each of them. Nevertheless, these were my first encounters with the fish in which my offerings had at least been obliged. And yes, there is *always* satisfaction in making a good cast with the right fly that a problem fish actually eats. I did not feel it as obsession turned its single-minded focus towards this new and even more powerful, elusive ghost of a fish, this fish with inordinately large, sentient and alien eyes. It is impossible to look at them, with those huge doll eyes, and believe they are from this world.

* * *

I would go to the cradle of saltwater angling, the Florida Keys, to learn all I could about the permit.

But first there was home, the land of concrete and steel, high concentrations of people, and the inescapable mirrors that reflect back the hard truth of one's physical being having been changed forever. The stranger's glance that becomes a double-take, and the slow giving up that is seeing oneself through their eyes rather than the more truthful, inward-looking eyes God has given each of us. I never bought into that, but my resolve to fight weakened. I began to drink too much to escape from myself and their eyes and judgment. After a while I simply got used to it. I would fish whenever financially possible, and get back to where I was judged only where it mattered to me anymore—with a fly rod in my hand, by guides, by fish, by God and by myself.

I was an unhappy and pathetic jester in the world of concrete and standard accomplishment. It was a living limbo. I moved to the closest salt water near my family, Galveston, where I could fish between fishing trips, and study fish in the classroom, too, at Texas A&M Galveston, as Marine Biology was not taught up at Baylor. I even got offered a job to write about fish and fishing. I took it.

CHAPTER VII

JEFFREY

We always had to get there before dawn on principle: the idea of the choicest areas, sure, but also for the pre-dawn tarpon bite and to watch the sun rise. It's S.O.P. anywhere in the Keys. Fast and blind on a plane in the dark, the *Waterlight* startled a four foot long houndfish near a spit of a key, and the beast accelerated into the air with irrational velocity and came to within six inches of impaling me through the neck. I could actually smell his fish slime as he flew underneath my nose before he reentered the water, on the other side and behind the hurtling skiff. I've never held one, but they must stink.

"If he'd spooked about a tenth of a second later, you'd be dead right now," Jeffrey said, over the full-throttle hum of the seventy horsepower outboard. "Imagine the coroner's expression and the obituary photos, Jim-bo." He smiled. Jeffrey's a photojournalist, in addition to being a guide.

"If it were quick," I said, "I'd be okay with that." I was in a good mood despite the fact that the night before I'd been kicked out of Sloppy Joe's bar on Duval Street before I had even had a chance to take a sip of the beer I'd just ordered; this, because they don't accept American Express and apparently don't like being asked if they do. Maybe the eye patch I had worn was simply too much—they must have presumed I was drunk and playing some pirate role, that it wasn't legitimate, and that I was not, in fact, saving them from an ugly sight.

Thanks to more recent surgery and a decent prosthetic, I do not feel the need for an eye patch anymore; but I will never forget those days when eyeball and socket irritation was just so bad I looked more a freak without a patch than with.

Kicking me out of Sloppy Joe's was doing me a favor though, as I'd gone to bed before twelve that Key West night, after briefly tucking my bruised tail between my legs and making my retreat to Pepe's, a Cuban place that is thankfully a little removed from the more superficial tourist places where no one knows that a bonefish is, for some, actually a reason to live, and not just something to be "done". They have excellent black bean soup, Pepe's, and they're not afraid of a guy with an eye patch.

Now, at nine in the morning, we could finally see well into the emerald green water. "You've paid your dues," Jeffrey said, from the poling platform of his Maverick. He is a blue-eyed, native Floridian guide, with a Spanish surname hailing of Europe. He's probably directly related to Christopher Columbus or Cabeza de Vaca because something stirred him in his youth and, at eighteen, he crossed the Atlantic in a small sailboat, alone.

"So I've paid my dues, huh?" I asked Jeffrey. "You mean mostly by just paying for trips and good guides," I finished. I had just blown an academic shot to passing ghost tarpon I had never even seen.

"That's bunk and you know it," he said. "Don't ever sell yourself short with a defeatist's attitude. You've put out the effort." He paused and scanned the water briefly. "And here *I* am, lazy guide."

He was running the electric motors with his toe switches as we crossed a turtle grass basin in pursuit of some rolling fish that had, Jeffrey theorized, just made it to the Marquesas Keys. "This'll be the first land mass they've run into since Cuba, so they're really happy," Jeffrey said.

Happy? I will not deny them this emotion. All one has to do is observe them for a while. They have mood swings like any other creature. And these fish, tarpon, have a primal tie to land, too: the river mouths, estuaries and marshes of land's margins along the tropical and subtropical zones of the Atlantic and Caribbean are feeding grounds and nursery havens to their offspring, and seeing land after days or even weeks of open sea might very well make them feel what we humans interpret as "happy"—they have, after all realized a major leg of their voyage. There are certainly worse places to be than the Marquesas if one is a tarpon, or an angler, for that matter.

The sea grass carpeted basin we crossed tapered up to an ochre flat, and snaking through the flat to the basin was a neon green finger channel—at some places it was an even deeper blue—that connected directly to the open sea. The happy tarpon were at the mouth of the channel as it opened into the basin, a hundred yards or so away from us now. They were rolling on the surface, inhaling and exhaling, and beginning to form a circular swimming pattern—a "daisy chain".

"Oh, yes," Jeffrey said. He had stopped the electrics and was gingerly picking up his push pole. "They're happy indeed. They're thinking about sex. When we get up to them, 'Bo, just cast to the oncoming edge of them."

When I figured the dynamic of the circle, I cast. This was 1991, the first year of Scientific Anglers Mastery Series Tarpon Taper Sinking fly line, and it is still to this day the quickest-shooting, farthest-casting fly line I've ever cast. It is so quick-loading when wet that putting the brakes on a presentation cast is often the order of the day. But this causes extreme turnover that can slap the water and scare fish out of their wits if one is not careful. I'd done just that earlier in the morning, so I was cautious now and my loop quickly but smoothly unrolled, placing the fly, a "Blue By You" of Jeffrey's, about three feet in front of oncoming tarpon traffic at the edge of the daisy chain.

"Strip it now, Jim," Jeffrey said.

On the second or third strip, something hit the fly and the impact was quickly transmitted up the tight line to my line hand. I struck, sweeping the rod sideways and pulling opposite with the line. Again and again, "driving the nail."

The fish reacted with a short blitzing run, a sudden stop and turn, and a charge at the boat. I stripped in slack line as fast as humanly possible, trying to restore tension and control, but this fish was just too fast. Then, a five foot barracuda propelled itself out of the water, into the air, and flew past my head. I froze on my feet. Fish were trying to kill me today.

The barracuda reentered the water and ran across the turtle grass basin, making my fly reel, a Pate Tarpon direct drive, sing.

"'Cuda thinks he's a tarpon," Jeffrey said. "This is bizarre."

No sooner had he said this when I felt the sudden, elusive pulling sensation that is the fly loosing from a fish's jaw, and a fish immediately past-tense. I reeled in a frazzled fly and shock tippet. We were quiet for a few moments.

"It's gonna' be a strange day," I said, staring into the water.

The daisy-chaining tarpon had fled the Marquesas Keys.

"Tide is coming up nicely now," Jeffrey said. "Let's go inside and look for permit."

We went inside Mooney Harbor, the large, shallow lagoon of the Marquesas which was, Jeffrey voiced, probably created by a meteor impact some sixty five million years in the past. It is certainly round enough in symmetry, has all sorts of magnetic activity at its periphery and does, as Jeffrey pointed out, lie along the same ballistic trajectory of acknowledged meteor impacts in Mexico's *Yucatán* and the Florida Everglades (4, Cardenas).

It came as no surprise to me that the Marquesas may be quite literally one of the very sites where many millennia of life's creatures were dealt the hand of inevitable finality, and where surviving life struggled to begin anew, in an essentially new world. The Marquesas and places like them do seem to harbor magic; they can certainly warp the way we perceive time: time can indeed stop here, as it does when a tarpon takes a fly or takes to the air; yet it can also move *very* quickly, as it does when said tarpon takes off on a long blitzing run and one suddenly notices the fly line is wrapped around one's leg, for instance.

This could be the very site of cataclysmic impact and climatic change so vast that dinosaurs were snuffed out and a furry little warm-blooded creature began to take a firmer hold, on land. The tarpon, somehow, survived the impact and the change it brought, as did sharks, bonefish, and other extant ancients, with their forms and genes intact. No wonder these fish are *tough*.

And yes, ultimately, a meteoric impact would offer an alternate explanation for the permit's very existence on this planet: they were not created nor did they evolve here, but instead were transported to Mother Earth via meteors—probably piloted the damned things—for the explicit purpose of befuddling the so-called minds of obsessive-compulsive anglers. The *Yucatán*, the Florida Everglades' outside Gulf region, and the Marquesas: geographic sites of meteor impacts that forever changed the face of the planet and, oh, yeah, they also *just happen* to be areas of high permit density. Coincidence? Facts happen first, and only then, after, are they called, "coincidences".

I present this, a tormented fly fisherman's hypothesis, to the scientific and angling communities as my argument that the permit is possibly, indeed, not of this world, and that permit fly rod anglers are not insane but are, in fact, the most qualified people on earth to deal with these aliens face-to-face; this, because we let them go unharmed after a little communication, always with a little "good-bye" and "thank you" kiss on the forehead. Extraterrestrial origin of the permit explains *everything*. They only talk to *us* ,when *they* choose to, and signal us that they want to talk by eating our *flies*.

If you are a permit angler you understand such insanity, as you, yourself, are so afflicted. If you are not, then the permit is just another fish.

As Jeffrey poled the *Waterlight* along the edge of a sea grass flat in the lagoon, we came upon a large live sponge inside a slight depression, surrounded by a circle of white sand that the dense green turtle grass bed had yielded its expansion to. I could see current flowing through the sponge's perfectly circular open mouth, inside of which was a large spiny lobster. A sea turtle, I believe a green sea turtle because it was green and elegant, hovered around the sponge, his head and large, soft brown eyes turning this way and that as he peered down into the mouth of the sponge, trying to figure out how to extract the lobster. He was completely unaware of the skiff and the two men on it, not twenty feet away. The turtle soon took on a desperate, frustrated look about him, and moved more frantically. We silently watched until Jeffrey quietly whispered, "Jim, I hate to interrupt this beautiful scene, but there's a permit way up on the flat *right now*, at one o'clock."

I looked up, out to the vast sandy and randomly sea grass-bedded flat. It was eerily quiet and the water's surface was completely flat. Directly under a blazing sun, yet highlighted by a background of dark gray cloud cover, the flat glowed a shock white and forest neon green in color, and there on it, some hundred yards away and precisely at one o'clock, I watched as a thin, black sickle blade suddenly appeared above the water's surface and violently thrashed to the side, silent in the distance, and kicked a narrow silver spike of water several feet straight up into the air. There was no sound as Jeffrey poled the skiff around the lobster and the turtle, and headed for the fish. Soon, the black tail appeared and kicked again, launching that vertical spike of water, and I made out the whole silvery body of a large permit.

"This is what's known as a 'spiking permit,' Jimbo," Jeffrey said. This fish was feeding with abandon. The wind began to pick up, steady and behind us, probably being sucked up by the approaching line of squalls that starkly highlighted the flat and the permit to our eyes. Things were ideal. *This could be it, this could really happen.* The fish cruised around and dipped down again, putting his tail into the air again.

"Okay, 'Bo," Jeffrey said. "No closer or he'll spook. Roll-cast now and go to him."

I did on command automatically, and about seven seconds later, my fly landed a few short feet in front of the now obviously large permit while his tail was still in the air. Right after impact, as I let the fly sink, the permit's tail disappeared below the water as he scooted forward to investigate. I was wired for the slightest touch through the tight fly line.

"He sees it on the bottom and he's not eating it. Strip it once, a twitch," Jeffrey said.

I followed orders, and watched the permit dip down for a second and then scoot off with a flurry, leaving puffs of sand suspended in the clear water. I had felt nothing through the fly line.

"Refusal," Jeffrey said, the air having left him. "Oh, God, he snubbed you cold."

I stripped my fly line in to make ready for another shot but the permit was now bolting off at an alien-speed clip down the flat, apparently insulted.

"Dammit, dammit, dammit," Jeffrey said as he came down off the casting platform with purpose. "Damn that Merkin. That was a great cast and a perfect presentation. If I'd made it, it would have been one of those rare, 'good job, Jeffrey, pat myself on the back', kind of casts." He was immediately at my side. "Give me that Merkin," he demanded. I handed it, still tied to my twelve pound leader, to him, and in one swift motion he put it to his mouth, severed the line with his teeth, and dashed the fly against the gunwale of his skiff, "Crack!" the lead eyes chimed on the fiberglass. "Damn that fly. Damn that Merkin. Let's try a McCrab."

"It's okay, Jeffrey," I said. "I'm used to that kind of rejection. And honestly, I don't know what I'd have to look forward to anymore if I caught one now."

He looked me in the eye and said, "I know *exactly* what you'd look forward to: catching *another* permit on a fly. *That's* what. On a fly that you tie yourself."

The black background that had highlighted that fish so had worked its way up near us and would cut us off from Key West and home if we did not skirt around it soon. Wind kicked up steadily. A bolt of lightning silently came down to the water, and its thunder hit us about ten seconds later—that's about two miles distance at the speed of sound at sea level. The air felt charged.

"When your hair stands on end, it's time to go," Jeffrey said. We headed home. On the way, during an anxious crossing of a confused and conflicted Boca Grande Channel that connects the Gulf of Mexico with the Straits of Florida and the Atlantic Ocean, the skies cleared and things began to look and feel promising for tomorrow. It was a vibe in the bones. Jeffrey suddenly laughed out loud and then leaned to me and said, over the snarling outboard, "You did it right, Jimbo: a man hasn't *done* Key West until he bags a tarpon on a fly and then, in the same day, goes and gets himself kicked out of Sloppy Joe's—with an eye patch no less. Then he makes a good shot at a huge permit the next day—damn that Merkin! I can't believe that shot. Man, I can't wait until tomorrow. Tell me, are you going to Sloppy Joe's again tonight, 'cause if you are, I wanna be there. See them try and mess with *my* angler. Man, I can't wait until tomorrow."

At the dock he introduced me to a tall and sinewy older gentleman who had waved to us as we pulled in and tied up at Garrison Bight Marina. His name was John Cole, and with a very brief time together he would have an impact on my life. He helped me to sell my first short story and, although I'd been published before, I'd never actually been paid with real money. It was a revelation to me. He gave me one of the greatest compliments a man can ever get by just saying, "You're fun to have around, kiddo."

So I did not catch a permit with a fly rod that day, or the next. Here's the way I look at it now: permit are like the grim reaper, death, and women—when it's your time, it's your time. It wasn't my time yet. And besides, looking at the most heated moments of the angling day, which is always very telling of the people involved, I had witnessed a stable man, Jeffrey, an alleged great angler of permit, verbally and physically abuse quite probably the single greatest fly ever created for permit on the face of the earth: the Dell Brown Permit Fly, the fabled Merkin. Big deal. Such is completely normal behavior. This is what a permit can do to a man in a moment of passion. Without that passion I would want no part of it; without that passion we would truly be insane. Or worse: we would be unworthy.

With something before me to strive for, I was *happy*.

One thing I hope never changes about Key West is this: if you absolutely just have to *land* a tarpon on a fly rod, book a day with a local guide in Key West.

CHAPTER VIII

GRACE

My friends and I met her at The Velvet Elvis, a dark bar with purple, florescent light-illuminated velvet paintings and an Elvis Presley theme, while at home in Houston between fishing trips and surgeries. What was different this time is that I, and not one of my friends, was the one who held her attention, and this, without any real effort on my part. It was purely a physical reaction. I looked at her: she was beautiful, lithe and graceful, with blue eyes and blonde hair tied up in a pony tail. My friends were on her like wolves and she looked around at them and smiled, used to the attention, and then her gaze settled on mine. She looked at my face through the darkness that surrounded the little round table as I sat down at it across from her, and I saw recognition in her eyes. She suddenly said, "Oh my God." And I immediately thought she had appraised the damage and simply had no social restraint or tact. I was, thankfully, wrong about this one.

She held me in her gaze, smiled seductively, and reached to her side and grabbed the sleeve of her friend's blouse. "Look at him," she said. Her friend, a big, warm brunette, turned and looked at me, raised her eyebrows and opened her mouth into a little "O" and said, "It's God! It's God! Oh my God!"

This is how I learned that some of the more insolent surgery nurses knew my father as "God".

"Why," I asked Grace, later, "do you call my father 'God'?"

"It's not that he has a God complex like some surgeons, Jim, and believe me some don't merit the huge egos they have. It's because he's good and he doesn't put up with any unnecessary bullshit from administrators or lazy nurses. And because, for God's sake, your name is 'Doggett'. Get it? D-O-G spelled backwards spells...?"

"Oh," I said. "Good. Otherwise I would have to thrash you for insulting my father."

She tilted her lovely almond shaped face up to the light and laughed, and put her warm hand into mine and squeezed. "Oh, Jim." she said. "You have no idea. But I would let your father operate on me."

I was lost. She should have just shot me.

My mind was occupied with Grace and I didn't think much about fly fishing until the relationship fell apart, the capitulation of which began almost immediately to the day that "marriage" came up in conversation, and not just in passing. A fishing guide brought me back around, again. Rick called from Islamorada with the free Gold Cup offer.

But first I had to do what I could to improve my damaged physical appearance. I had delayed the scheduling of further necessary reconstructive surgeries long enough. I soon was reminded why I had delayed them so long: the pain of re-breaking old injuries that are healed.

* * *

I awoke hearing Grace being paged over a speaker in the recovery room. But no, she had not come back to me. She was there merely doing her job. My father stood over me and gave me some ice chips. I never saw her again. Was I just a notch on her bedpost? Had I been used? Well, there are few creatures more physically aware and compassionate than a young surgery nurse is, and I had had a damned good time. I will not complain about getting to love someone. So what's the big deal? Shut up and go fish with your broken heart. There are more fish in the sea.

* * *

PART TWO

CHAPTER IX

M.G.

Bay of the Ascension of Christ, Mexico, summer, 2000:

Acres upon acres of white coral sand and limestone marl are covered with three to four feet of warm, clear salt water that reflects a translucent emerald green under the midday sun. The green is chlorophyll in phytoplankton—diatoms, algae and the like—as the very water is alive. White through neon green is inescapably everywhere, drawing and warmly feeding the eye. A very few small sand spits, whirled and shoaled by tidal ebb and flow, rise near the surface where individual mangrove shoots have taken hold. These ambitious plants are the only visible interruptions to the expanse of green florescence.

If I were to look up I would see a moist blue summer sky with a few random, puffy white cotton balls of presently benign cloud, the high sun patient with the afternoon ahead to evaporate but also laden some with heavy moisture from the sea in a tug of war of water, wind and heat. But if one looks up for more than a few seconds while hunting with a fly rod one is being the irresponsible cad, as the fish are in the water.

The pain I perpetually seek to escape with every legal means has been slowly building, originating at the mid-spine in a dull, persistent heat. It is a knotted fist of compression that courses down the spine and expands out through the thoracic cavity with reaching, throbbing fingers. Pressure and heat. Vision and thought will become progressively funneled through a narrowing tube of focus. Inevitably, these sensations will coalesce and become their own living beast, effectively replacing me. I concentrate my focus into and through the green water as we drift along. I see the slight wavy undulations of the vast sandy bottom, and my eye, hungry for variation, looks forward to the arrival of each rare, white rising dome of deposit that surrounds the lonely mangrove shoots as we float upon them. So attuned to visual detail, I become lost in it; thought is removed and reactionary predation can take its place. This is of great benefit for the critical moments when the kind of visual interruption that moves of its own volition appears.

I quickly glance over my shoulder to check that my stripped-out fly line isn't attempting to breed with the unbridled bow line below the skiff's casting platform again, and catch their sign on the water out of the corner of my eye: a pair of surface wakes approaching from behind, at our six o'clock. The wakes do not wander in their path; they appear driven by tandem torpedoes in perfect parallel. Such purposeful sign indicates fish going from "A" to "B" in a hurry and not dilly-dallying to feed. Their eyes will be especially alert to any movement, be it from predator or prey, and their other senses similarly wired. These fish are opportunists—especially in the eat-or-be-eaten marine environment—and, like children, they sometimes reveal an overpowering curiosity by taking even unlikely opportunities into their mouths. There would be little success in angling if it were not for this endearing trait.

I now make out a long, narrow, very defined black streak immediately in front of each V-wake, which instantly distinguishes these fish as permit, *Trachinotus falcatus* .

I feel the familiar heated surge of adrenalin in my chest as my heart first rises with heightened anticipation and then drops to my belly with lowered expectation. I can forget about *these* fish being overcome with curiosity and eating anything that is not positively identified as a legitimate food item first. As a solo angler, I spend close to two hundred days each year hunting shallow salt waters with a fly rod in my hand, and yet it still happens every single time—with the permit more than any other species. Such physical epinephren rush coupled with a deep enigmatic mind-job pushes buttons in my brain; it opens receptors that, once initially activated with that first fix more than a decade ago, must be fed on a regular basis. I noticed back then that, at such times, and even at times when action is only highly likely, I become suddenly free of all physical pain.

About three seconds have passed since I spotted the fish.

"Fish at our six, Eduardo," I say to my guide, who's controlling the skiff's drift with his push pole in the stern. Eduardo turns and looks behind the boat, briefly scans then nods his head, and quickly turns back to face me, shaking his head: *don't cast right now or you'll nail me, or your friend eating the lobster sandwich in the middle of the boat.*

He doesn't know me. It is our first day together on the water, which always seems a period of break-in for guide and angler as a team. We've got about ten seconds before the fish draw even with the skiff, but I do not want to miss the head-on approach shot, which would be a sacrilege.

And a fly rod is the only thing in my life I can still control.

"I've got a shot," I say, and roll cast the line out safely over the water, over my opposite shoulder. I shoot a little line out when the rod unloads, then come back with a back-cast, using the water tension on the fly line to load the rod. I shoot more line behind me, then come forward with the bending rod and halt it with the thumb and the rod aimed right at the target—the path of the fish—and unload the cast. The loop of fly line that now contains all of the energy of the rod travels quickly out and progressively unrolls, turning over the leader and fly about ten feet in front of the lead, advancing permit. I see a big drop of water rise an inch or two into the air where the fly—a heavy lead-eyed, #2 tan yarn crab fly that Eduardo tied—enters the water. All takes about four seconds.

"Hmmmm...," Eduardo, with raised eyebrows, remarks.

Such a heavy fly almost invariably makes a noisy stage entrance; so, I trust, the fish already see it as it dives to the bottom—which is what crabs, in a desperate attempt to hide under the sand, are purported to do when they sense a pair of approaching, crab-loving permit.

The lead surface wake widens and breaks up as the fish slows, dips down, and follows the sinking fly. All I see through the water is the long, narrow black streak of her back getting longer as the fish angles nose-down. Then she rises back up and proceeds forward again. I strip the fly once, in a short little hop, to get her partner's attention. She glances and snubs it coldly, also, then speeds ahead to catch up with her partner. I strip the line back in as quickly as I can.

"Refusal," Eduardo says, from his perch on the stern bench. "El doble."

Now the fish are approaching a parallel with the boat, some fifty feet out, proceeding on their trek undaunted. My eye is irrevocably drawn to the defining visual trait of a permit moving in profile over a light sand bottom: their powerful black tail, looking like a sideways "Y", beats quickly and purposely back and forth behind the black stripe that tops the fish's dorsal fin and back. It is this cyclic motion that rivets me with a feeling of immediacy and anxiety each time I see it.

As they draw even with the boat, I see their enormous, sentient, doll-like eyes. And once I can make out the eyes, I've got the whole fish: these are garbage-lid sized permit of twenty to thirty pounds. Their broad, pearlescent silver sides reflect the white bottom like liquid mirrors. I cast to the side, over the water throughout the stroke again rather than through the boat, and lead their path several feet on the presentation. The fly sinks well in front of them—I see it diving head-first to bottom, a near-perfect intercept, and see the lead fish stop on top of the fly and dip down to it. I see a puff of sand flower in front of the fish's nose as she smells it and—feeling nothing through the tight line—refuses.

"Strip it, just twitch it," Eduardo says, and I oblige. I see the permit tilt back up, and she and her partner move onward again. My heart is in my throat. *She might have eaten it, what with the puff of sand, but I felt nothing.* My mind begins a cycle of conflict but I quickly quell it. *Not now.*

The permit are showing us their kicking backsides, slightly accelerating as they depart, yet still unwavering on their course.

Eduardo shrugs his shoulders and says, "They not eat that, they eat nothing."

I'm not through with them yet.

I picture perfect form and a straight-line rod-path in my mind as I cast full-out, my body rocking quickly with each line-haul and rod-stroke, shooting line after each as the rod craves it, and then I let a deep drive go, my thumb and the stout, unloading rod aimed at an intercept point an obscene distance out in front of the skiff for the only presentation possibility: an angled-away leading shot, one overtaking the fish's departing direction. A long shot, but every shot at a permit is a long shot.

All I see is my pointing-elbow-shaped loop of fly line flying fast, out to the target; I hear the sweet snaking zip-song of the running line as it flies through the rod guides, pulled out by the airfoil loop, and then feel and hear the "slap" as the tail end of the fly line impacts the rod between the reel and the first stripping guide. In the distance I see line and leader sharply unroll, fall, and lay out straight on the water, the terminal end of it and the fly in front of the fish some four to six feet. Things are looking up.

Eduardo lets out a whistle, and I feel a warm rush of humility and pride fill my chest. Every hair on my body tingles at this, my guide's simple acknowledgment of the work I have done to hone a skill.

We watch as the lead fish actually angles off course to the fly and stops. Her black scimitar of a tail does not, however, rise up to indicate at least a close inspection. No, she's just suspended there in apparent indecision.

"Strip it, Jim," Eduardo says.

I strip the fly line once, pulling the fly off the bottom for a hop.

"Again," Eduardo says. I fight ingrained technique learned in the Florida Keys, where to move a properly presented crab fly is anathema. But there is one Golden rule I always try and heed: always listen to your guide. I move the fly. We watch as the fish angles back to its original course and moves on, its patient partner in wing man formation. They've had enough.

Less than a minute has passed since I first spotted the fish. Three good shots and no eats. It's the shots that count, I know, as no human can control what a permit thinks or does at any given time. *Yes, Jim, be thankful; for it could have been very ugly indeed.* I would soon see a man literally fold up and almost cry while facing a permit and find it impossible to hold this one act against him.

In the suddenly oppressive calm, the inflammation around the crushed thoracic vertebra brings me back into my body. I slowly lay down on the casting platform. *Ten minutes lying down and I'll be good for another hour, so deal with it. You're on your stage of choice.*

Supine, I look up into the blue sky and feel the relief I know is only transitory slowly flow around like a mist. I resolve to increase my physical therapy exercise—which is just lifting iron at unusual angles—to four times a week instead of only two or three times. The regularity of it is good for the mind; knowing one is doing all he can is as important as the building of muscle around compromised bones and joints is. Fishing time goes up in direct proportion, and bitching time goes down.

"M.G.," I call to my boat mate. "Beer me, *ahora mismo* ('this instant' in Spanish, which M.G. does not speak)." I have been saying little Spanish quips all day.

Eduardo smiles and laughs. I turn my head to look at M.G. He's furrowing his brow and shaking his head. *Uh oh.* He fetches a brown Carta Blanca from under the ice in the cooler, opens it with the bottle opener mounted in the bilge, and walks forward and slaps it into my hand.

"Stop that Spanish shit *'ahora mismo'* or this is the last beer you'll ever drink," he quietly says. He's a quick study.

"If only that were true, my friend," I smile to him. "But you're right and I'm sorry. Speaking in a foreign tongue around anybody is the greatest insult and I didn't mean it. I was just trying to impress Eduardo, here."

He stops in his tracks, his mouth hanging in apparent disbelief. "Jesus, Jim," M.G. says, shaking his head in frustration. "Can't you see you've already done that?" He points to where I had last cast, opens his palms up to the blue sky, and then drops them to his sides in a slap. He turns his back to me, sighs, and slowly scans the emerald flat. "You scare me sometimes," he says.

And the humility and pride I had been feeling, warm and glowing in my chest, curdles with confusion and shame.

I drink the cold beer, supine, and look up into the blue sky to see an osprey flying low and fast with a fish in its talons. *Is it a bonefish? They're certainly plentiful and small enough for an osprey here.* She screams a high-pitched chirping cry to us. I follow the raptor and see her land in a tangled nest atop a tall butternut mangrove in a dense mott. She chows on the fish, unknowingly mocking the silly man with the $700.00 fly rod.

I think once again to myself that if I catch a permit, maybe everything will be all right and I can die complete. This is a lot to put on a fish's narrow shoulders, I know. But a permit is a lot of fish.

CHAPTER X

MARK

The next day, five p.m.:

Three tired, seemingly unfettered young sports left the tied off skiffs at the lagoon and loped along a groomed white sand trail lined with tall coconut palm trees, stocky palmetto shrubs, and Australian pines. I hobbled along behind them with my four rinsed fly rods and the Playmate cooler full of Mexican beer and ice. I was a walking symbol of myself. The hot sun, broken by the palm canopy overhead, flashed my friends with bright mottled light as they advanced ahead of me. They slowed as they hit the soft, subtle rise of the dune before they broke out onto the blazing white of open beach. I paused at mid-dune and watched them as they bounced on one foot first and then the other as they shed their wading booties. They made no pause on the hot coarse sand but quickly crashed into the clear, gently rolling Western Caribbean surf. They stood, floated and swam in a painter's palette of ochre, turquoise and green.

I hung my rods in the shaded screened porch of my cabin of the week, and pulled four Carta Blancas from the bottom of the ice in the cooler. I popped the tops by placing the bottom of my Bic lighter snugly between the cap and my index finger, which was curled tightly around the bottle neck. A quick "whack," to the top half of the lighter and you're in business. I nestled the bottles back safely in the ice and moseyed on down with them to join my friends in the surf who, at the sight of the coldest beer in Mexico, were revitalized like pit bulls for an instant.

The eighty-five degree water quickly cooled our browned and reddened skin, and its buoyancy relaxed knotted muscles and over-taxed bones and joints. A wave of relief overcame all as we suspended in cool aquamarine space. Sips from the iced beer brought a completeness to the day, and I felt a smile wash over me by uncontrollable reflex. I looked around at my friends, now arranged in a floating circle: they were all smiling, too.

This was our ritual at day's end.

I looked over to my angling partner that day: Mark was bobbing like a cork at the drop-off of the sandbar, and absolutely glowing with contentment and sunburn.

"Slam, Jim," he boomed aloud, and waded over to me with his big pink palm outstretched for a high-five.

"Slap!" my palm met his.

"Super Slam, actually," I said. "That's a bonefish, tarpon, permit AND snook all in one day."

"Our guide caught that permit, though, Jim," Mark quietly said.

My face slackened at this sudden confession. Mark had been boasting his catch to our friends since we had regrouped at the dock.

"What's wrong, Jimbo?"

"I honestly don't know. I think I need another beer."

"Set me up, too, would you?"

As I waded to the beach and the waiting cooler, I grew angry with my friend's selective honesty. "He tests my loyalty to him with this because, of course, I was in the same skiff, right next to him, at crime's commission," I said to myself. I sighed and shook my head.

It had been ugly. After some frustrated attempts by Mark to deliver the fly to permit, Eduardo had asked him to cast his tan rag head crab fly to a completely vacant, white sand channel between two huge turtle grass beds, and to just let the fly sit on the bottom. He did so and, fully two minutes later, a small school of permit had come swimming along the channel to the fly's exact location, whence one desperado had promptly inhaled it and self-set the hook as it turned to swim away. The permit weighed around fifteen pounds. A very nice fish.

I had been respectful of Eduardo's ability to find—and apparently train—wild fish from that moment on. But even more cunning was his sense of reading a client: he knew what buttons to push to get that permit and the Super Slam, and that Mark would be a willing pawn to the manipulated catch.

Wading back to the beach, I came to a sad realization: the guides must do this kind of thing all too often to bag fish for the expectant, yet mediocre caster. A couple of decades of guiding the wrong kind of "sport" would make such a practice almost occupational necessity, as this is still the third world, where a guide's salary is the stipend and tips are everything. To his mind, Eduardo was merely doing his job, and superhumanly, at that. "He obviously does better with the casualties than I do," I said to a brown pelican on the beach who was watching me. I looked back into the clear surf and followed a dark, watermelon-sized shape as it paralleled close to shore, towards my friends—a big snook, or maybe a cubera snapper.

So, Mark had just betrayed himself with his insecurity-based posturing to build his esteem in the eyes of his friends. I imagined one domino falling down, hitting another; that one hit another and on and on. A man's character was made up of those dominoes laying on the ground. *Maybe it gets easier after a couple fall down. Maybe I'm taking this all too seriously. Of course I am not: this is fishing. How can he do this to himself?*

Mark is a decent caster; he just hasn't spent the time to hone it all to an edge, to sharpen his loops with a quick and decisive rod stop and speed it all up with his line hand to get the fly delivered to the fish quickly. Dedication is all that is lacking. That others did not make such a commitment and yet, to all observation, demanded the rewards, baffled me.

As I pulled two amber bottles from the ice, I felt resignation make an attempt to wash over me. "So this is the way it's going to be," I said to myself. *Honesty only when it's convenient.*

But there was one other integral issue I could not look beyond. I could not be passive-aggressive about it, either, and settle for just sliding a couple of dead hermit crabs down to the bottom of his fly rod carrying case with a little Zap-a-Gap super glue (a thousand and two uses). Better to be more direct. I returned to the healing waters.

"Thanks for handing me the rod that time," I said to Mark. "That was big of you."

"Oh, that wind was giving me bloody hell," he smiled. "There was absolutely no way I could reach that fish, and I knew you could. Great cast, by the way," he said, and then shook his head. "I can't believe he didn't eat your fly."

This was a strategic complement.

"That's how permit normally behave, Mark" I said. "By the way, did you recognize that fly rod?" I felt a tinge of fear and anticipation in my chest as I asked, but the irony was too much for me to ignore.

"What, your awesome permit rod?" my friend asked.

"Yup."

He mulled that over for a minute and said, "No, why?"

This was the wrong answer.

"That's my 'repaired' (I made quotation marks with my fingers in the air for emphasis), 1990 model 1090 RPLX Sage, undeniably the best permit fly rod ever made. And they stopped making them years ago. You remember: it's the one you obliterated at my bay house this May."

A blush appeared through Mark's sunburn and he fidgeted. "Hmm," he said, averting his bulging gray eyes.

"I'm still out a hundred bucks for that shattered rod, the same—excuse me, not *quite* the same—rod that just bagged a permit for you."

"I'll be damned, Jim," he said. "Well they did a great job, didn't they? Casts like a dream."

"Yeah. Small world, huh?"

And I watched the familiar change sweep over my friend. His features hardened and the defensive walls rose back up again, barring all who would dare try to look inside and call him out.

Damn you is right, I thought to himself. *I don't know how to help you, and right now I don't want to, anyway.* I downed the beer before it got any warmer and waded back to the beach and the waiting cooler.

I knew I had just eaten the cost of my now-bipolar permit fly rod.

"I want to fish alone," I said to the brown pelican on the beach. "Forever alone."

The very next day, through our fourth party on the trip, a traveling fly shop owner, Mark would indeed buy what may have been the actual, last unused and unsoiled 1090 RPLX in existence—for himself.

I was so incensed I was incapable of realizing that Mark had actually given me a rare gift that day on the water. He had had the humility, sportsmanship and, ultimately, the practicality to surrender the bow to me, so that I could take a shot at a permit he could not reach. A small sacrifice? No. Coming from Mark it was huge, a legitimate "breakthrough" moment. I see it as his true character fighting its way through the insurmountably pure narcissism he displays when he is center stage, his often dormant, giving nature and his respect and observance of sportsmanship saving the day, conceding the bow to the better athlete and in that moment eclipsing all the weaknesses he may indeed have. A shot at a permit is the greatest gift anyone can give to someone like me.

There are too many anglers who are of the mindset that if they themselves cannot reach a fish, then they will deny others the opportunity, even bitch it by trashing it.

Nonetheless, friendship with Mark usually seems to be a verb, a constant state of bafflement and stretching the boundaries of forgiveness. But it is friendship. A fly rod, a material thing, can be replaced—or at least substituted; a friend, complete with albatross and kryptonite around the neck though he may be, cannot. He's a pill, God love him.

* * *

Of course to a drinker of alcohol, whether the drinking is justified as pain management, psychological damage control, or just the old-fashioned mind-numbing of reality, the inevitable result is that, done often enough, the drinker's body and mind do more than become merely "accustomed to it" at some point: they become addicted to it. Though I had never read the possibility of this event occurring on the label of any bottle, I now knew that it indeed had happened to me. It does not "run in my family". It was the direct result of my behavior: my drinking it chronically to excess because of my inability to cope with deep, irretrievable loss. Complicating the issue with other reasons and conditions merely avoids facing the truth and taking responsibility for it.

So today, with my new, bi-polar fly rod, the manipulated permit and the selective *bloviating* of my friend Mark, I had endured too much irony for one day. I drank my fave: twelve-year-old Johnnie Walker Black Label scotch with a splash of soda, copper in color and biting, grainy-bitter in taste, very much alone despite all the talking and congratulating—there are typically only six or seven Super Grand Slams on fly tackle each year at the lodge, and it's a *very* big deal. During the T-shirt ritual, I ruminated in the bitterness of the drink and of my heart. The bonefish, tarpon and snook are not particularly difficult for even the neophyte to luck into with a good guide. It is the permit, this one infuriating fish, that is highly unpredictable and hesitant to take a fly. This fish seems to choose the angler and not the other way around, as it is in a normal world. As a direct result of the fish's unique personality there exists an elite and unspoken Permit Club. When I began pursuing the fish, there were a few hundred people in the world who'd taken a permit with a fly rod and thus were accorded membership. New fly patterns and techniques over the ensuing years had radically increased the number of inductees. But, because of the very nature of the fish itself, there would always exist a much larger and infinitely quieter Sans Permit Club. Such a brotherhood no longer offered me any solace; for, over the course of my twelve year quest, a feeling of unacknowl-edged entitlement, a quiet indignation, had crept in and overshadowed any feelings of belonging. My mind began to swim in a vicious circle, con-suming itself in a tightening loop. I was a time bomb. Anglers on jinxed, career-length permit jags are not to be trifled with. A waiter brought Mark a special slice of cake with a sparkler, ablaze and shooting sparks, stuck in its middle. There was applause. I fell deeper.

There were of course the angling buffoons who, through a perverted sequence of events the likes of which airline crashes and nuclear meltdowns result, luck into a permit blindly. *God himself seems to have touched these people,* I thought to myself, *and yet, because of the almost accidental nature of the catch, these people cannot ever have any real appreciation for the fish, the event. There is no real meaning to it. They have not suffered, gone through the pain.* There it was: a glimmer.

But it was impossible for me to fully realize that it was this very real pain and travail of the pursuit that was the true gift, the real reward of such a single-minded quest. I simply had to see the other side of it, had to hold this precious fish in my hands. Only then could I appreciate how the "lucky" people never attained such powerful emotions, how they were de-nied the gift by their luck. The burning fact is that the Pain of Worthiness Earned is denied untold thousands of anglers by the sheer cunning of that deadliest creature ever to carve the surface of the flats with push pole and fly rod: the professional flats guide.

Instead of at least pitying the lucky, I saw them as simple undeserv-ing buffoons, circus clowns with no ability, no discipline and no proper reverence for the quarry and the game. They were the New Fly Fisher-men, products of the new millennium that had jumped into the blender of commercialization and come out in shockingly trendy angling garb with stratospheric expectations that frightened me, and surely puzzled the world's finest fish and flats guides. *Digital permit,* I thought. *The goal is achieved before it is even a goal. I'm a dinosaur surrounded by rats. Perhaps I should just roll over and let them eat me. Maybe I'm taking this all too seriously. Nope.* At thirty-five years of age, I was still running on testosterone and booze, and could not look back with hind-sight and remember that I, too, had started at the beginning. But I had started with a cherishing of all innocent life that is gained only by having one's own crushed, and snuffed out. I cannot, nor do I want to give them that, because of the cost.

I drank to drown the charlatans, the false-anglers and their manipulative guides that had taken residence in my troubled mind. I drank to their drowning as they slept their corrupted and conscious-less sleep of lies. I drank, as John Cole wrote and, later, actually said to me at his Key West Angler's Club, "with silence and determination." As I looked into the vaporous amber liquid, I thought I actually heard John speak these very words to me in his New Englander drogue. I quickly scanned the bar, confused.

I'd just had my first auditory hallucination.

Booze and permit angling are a bad combination.

* * *

CHAPTER XI

ALFONSO

The last day:

Modern medicine kept me going. A Prilosec ™ anti-acid reflux cap-sule each morning kept Hydrochloric acid from both eating a whole in my stomach and rising into my throat. On taking it I always felt that I could continue my alcoholic gastrointestinal abuse for at least one more day. There was great security in that. I swallowed the capsule with cold black coffee—which was definitely pushing it—back in my room and knew that, after imposing my will upon that first fish or two of the day, I'd be ready for breakfast beer.

From the water, the southern border of *La Bahía Campechen* is seemingly an abrupt and lengthy wall of impenetrable mangrove forest; but there is at least one break in the twisted marine roots that opens into an inner sanctum: saltwater lakes that are *almost* entities apart from the main, farther removed from the open bay and Caribbean, like I had become from the rest of humanity. To the south, these lakes open up to the flats of another bay, the Bay of the Ascension of Christ, *La Bahía de la Ascensión del Christo.*

The bottom of the small shallow creek channel we navigated to get to her is dense, sharp oyster. Alfonso watched the prop's progress, his face occupied with concern. I stood and looked down at the prop, and saw that it was aluminum—easily shattered. Alfonso glanced quickly at me and then looked back into the churned water. *There's plenty of it and I know what I'm doing,* he exuded. I smiled at his cockiness, young guide.

We finally cleared the oyster and got on a plane, then flew around quick switch-backs in the mangrove channel. As we rounded one last S-curve, flashes of panicked pink and crimson suddenly filled the air and scattered immediately ahead of the boat: a pod of Roseate Spoonbills, shocked at the sudden materialization of a rat skiff into their peaceful world, fled their feeding ground at the mouth of the lagoon. This was a quieter world. With less direct tidal ebb and flow, the water was slightly tannin-stained around the mangrove roots, like a weak tea, from decaying detritus.

This is quintessential juvenile tarpon habitat. A school of maybe a hundred or so young tarpon had been here, in a huge turtle grass bottomed basin, for five days straight. These were fifteen to twenty five and thirty pound fish, five to ten year-old tarpon that were approaching the time when they would leave the relative safety of the mangrove sanctuary for at least part of their lives to swim in the open bays and, soon, even venture out into the Western Caribbean, and the Gulf of Mexico.

And we had found the tarpon here, like tarpon everywhere, by taking advantage of their wonderful evolutionary trait, their swim bladder, the buoyancy organ that is also a functional lung : our guide shut the motor down and we sat quietly at first light, listening for the sighing sounds as the fish rolled on the surface, exhaled, and then inhaled fresh air, like submarine horses.

Today was the sixth day and we heard nothing. We drifted and listened.

These fish had become the morning ritual for each of us. Each had played the game of silver leaps and runs from start to finish over this fish bowl in the lagoon, and each had brought a marine denizen that shared the air he himself breathes to hand—each except for M.G., I suddenly realized. Even though it was my time up on the casting platform, I looked over to my friend to offer him the first shot. Sitting there at my shoulder, stoic and loyal, was this man who, when he'd heard I'd lost an eye at school, had walked around for a full day with one of his own eyes covered.

I was about to give him my fly rod when Alfonso said, "Tarpon gone, Mister Jim. Grab your snook rod. Good fish in the next laguna."

Priorities.

* * *

Lime green met tea-green as overhanging mangrove leaves reached out to claim more of the cove, the red-brown reaching roots still, however, allowed a navigable opening for the skiff. This would be overgrown within a few years through succession, as land is created from salt water, sand and root; yet this only temporary, too, as the next hurricane will reclaim it for the marine water world once again, ripping the conquering plants apart, down to their very roots, twisting and killing their life-giving green. Acres of it are simply ripped up and rolled like tumbleweeds to gray and rot. But the cycle continues, as surviving edges of mangrove begin the decades-long process of reclamation and succession. Released seedlings, floating mangrove "pencils", sprout roots wherever they touch new ground.

What a hopeful plant, I thought to myself as I stared into the roots of the red mangrove, transfixed. So twisted, confused and impossibly tangled were these roots, growing on any substrate they can find like metastasizing cancer. I felt their life mirrored my own mind's journey along the vicious cycle-trail of alcohol: progressively warped synapses formed distorted ideas and leapt to paranoid conclusions, and expanded their deluded territory. Yet I was starkly aware that the ceaseless pounding of alcohol into my body would eventually, as a simple matter of course, purge my consciousness of most any thought at all, twisted or otherwise, like a hurricane sweeping through the mind. But the mind, unlike the mangrove, cannot ever truly regenerate. When brain tissue dies it is gone forever. There would be only barren sea with no mangrove seedling to start anew again, in the end. I was suddenly aware of this failed analogy as I stood on the platform of the skiff.

"What a buzz-kill," I said to myself.

It was the fly rod I held in my hand that kept a panic attack at bay—that, and the fat-headed snook that was peeking out from the mangled roots before me. Sharp adrenaline focus instantly eradicated moribund musings, my sudden, clear realization of the inevitable. The snook faced outward with the falling tide, awaiting the hapless bait fish, shrimp and crabs that could not cling to something or bury themselves. It is this expectation on the part of the snook that provides an opportunity for the angler which he can bank on time and time again. This was a welcome respite between hunts for the neuroses-wrought permit. *Hey, isn't fishing supposed to be fun, after all?* I thought to myself.

The rod is held at an angle to the side in the cast, and the stroke is up on the back cast and down on the forecast. I hit it hard on the presentation, twisting up with the thumb at the last microsecond. This skipped the fly and terminal end of the leader off the water, and flipped them up under the overhanging canopy of mangrove leaves and branches, right into the faces of the expectant snook. They simply would not eat a fly presented at the edge of clearing when they were inside the canopy—it had to be in their domain. When shown this homage the snook took with abandon, as if they had been patiently waiting for a worthy opponent to play a game with.

I stripped the green and white Lefty's Deceiver fly and a big dark log swam out from deeper in the roots, opened a gray-white mouth and socked the fly, then turned ninety degrees. I stopped him in his tracks before he could turn another ninety degrees and dive for cover. I pulled the snook from the safety of the roots, out into the open water. A feeling passed through my chest and I seized it, pulling it back.

"M.G.," I said. "Want to play this fish?"

"Absolutely," he answered, and then walked up to me and took the rod. "But if it were anyone other than you, Jimbo, I'd be ashamed."

And I felt a weight I didn't know existed as it left my shoulders, and a heavy cloud as it lifted away from my soul.

Aside from tossing a lure with a spinning rod only once or twice when prodded, my noble and quiet friend had taken to enjoying the fishing only vicariously. He never asked to cast and seemed quite happy. Such humility was especially surprising since M.G. was a natural athlete who took to everything—everything but a fly rod, that is. *Finally facing something he could not immediately master must have been frustrating*, I thought. *He must be a mature adult human being.*

I lay down on the middle bench and watched him play the snook. Alfonso brought me a beer, and we watched and smiled. I felt a peace I hadn't felt in years. We stayed in the cove until the tide stopped falling, and the snook suddenly ceased the game as if a switch had been thrown.

* * *

With the tide at low the oyster-bottomed channel was too shallow for the outboard, so Alfonso locked the motor up and guided the skiff out with his push pole. I took my heavy sunglasses off and cleaned the lens with a dry cotton towel. I smiled. A few years ago I was about to wipe a fogged rifle scope lens with a paper towel when I felt a hand stop mine. I looked up at my mentor Chuck Scates, Texas flats guide, who was shaking his head slowly as he said, "Never use anything that comes from a tree on optics—here's a towel." And I took it and said, "But cotton's from a plant, too, Chuck." He shook his head again, smiled and said, "Grasshopper, grasshopper. Cotton's from a bush, not a tree. Bush good, tree bad."

We headed back north, towards the *Boca*, or mouth, that connects the massive lagoon system with the Western Caribbean, feeding it and draining it with the tide. In the heat of summer the water coming in, at eighty-two to eighty-four degrees (my thermometer had developed an air pocket in the fluid, and I could not be sure exactly), was at least five degrees cooler than that water which had been draining out. Interestingly, we'd been seeing and catching bonefish in the lagoon well into the afternoons when water temperatures were as high as ninety degrees. I theorized it must be a population adaptation, as bonefish typically prefer water much cooler. That they'd endure such heat rather than stay in the cool sea is testimony to both the richness of prey and the comparative safety they must have in these *Yucatán* bays. While the bonefish may merely have tolerated it, the permit seemed to absolutely thrive in the heat. I was convinced these fish would remain to frolic in the sun-heated, almost body-temperature waters long after I had literally cooked my brain, just to spite me.

We flew to the end of the peninsula of densely foliated land that jutted into the bay and paralleled the channel of the *Boca*, where the first cool, incoming tide waters washed over a small sea grass flat that tapered up from the channel's deeper edge. Alfonso clicked the motor up and grabbed his push pole, and just then I saw a lone permit, once peacefully working the edge of the flat in the deep grass at the drop off, as he bolted in fear ahead of the skiff, back through the *Boca* channel to the ocean, his black stripes of back and tail and his bulbous water bulge rocketing over the tops of sea fans and green and brown gorgonian sponges that looked like huge heads of lettuce. A rush of sudden panic filled my chest. My breathing accelerated. I felt a clammy chill. A picture formed in my mind:

I'm isolated by choice here—have been for months or years—and I'm living on a fermented, one hundred proof concoction I make of coconuts and bonefish slime—the sebaceous, protective secretion that liberally covers both the bonefish and the angler who catches and holds him. I'm standing naked at sunset, up to my knees in gin clear water, holding a live permit in my hands; I bite it behind its narrow, tall head, chomp down to the backbone, snap its neck in my jaws, and feel it quiver in death as I drink its coppery, fishy blood. I'm standing here covered with sand fleas, mosquitos, and the blood of a fish I love and have just murdered, churning in an inescapable madness all alone.

I could not shut out images like this from forming in my mind. They were commonplace now, without focused thought, forming like the words of a response to a question in a casual conversation form in the mind of the listener—a person who in this case is impatient and interrupts the speaker with his presumed answer. I could no longer control my own thoughts, as they simply raced ahead of me.

"God, help me," I whispered to myself, and reached to my ten weight under the bungee chord that secured the rod butts to the stern bench.

Alfonso, watching me, said, "Let's do bonefish, Jim."

I picked up my seven weight, instead.

"Thank you, God," I said aloud.

Bonefish are like cherished pets to me. They inspire loyalty. And as each individual dog or cat is unique in some way, so it seems to be with each of the hundreds of bonefish I've somehow managed to meet: circumstances of terrain, the take and fight, are always a little different; and sometimes, from one fish to the next, they can and do behave as if they were of a different species altogether. One constant with all bonefish is that first, blazing run of panic (unless one is a killjoy and, if close to the bonefish and using heavy tippet, he locks down on the line right at the take, denying the fish his momentum and denying himself the earned gift of the run). Depending on local fishing and other human pressures, she can be uneducated and easy or, as in the Florida Keys, extremely wary—even jaded and cynical. Yet no matter her disposition, another giving trait of the bonefish is that she will still oblige the proper presentation of the proper fly at the proper time. There is always this hope. And they give all of themselves. Arriving to hand completely spent, they remain absolutely motionless—especially if held upside down—until their resuscitation and release. No other fish has so rewarded every effort of my heart, and soothed my troubled mind.

I believe that the bonefish, though, like the tarpon, a species extant for millennia, would probably not be any different if she were, say, the product of reverse-engineering: God makes Man and the fly fisher-Man, and he is given the grace to design the ultimate fly rod quarry and, naturally, he comes up with the bonefish.

This flat, so near the mouth of the Caribbean, is more dynamic than most: its marine visitors represent more of the food chain, and each successive member is keenly aware his chief predator may be close behind him. The bonefish are the most obviously nervous, and must really feel they're in a conundrum when faced with *just so much tempting food to eat.*

Alfonso poled the skiff off the channel edge and staked the boat high up on the flat, over thick turtle grass beds in about a foot of water. We did not wait long before a school of some twenty bonefish worked up onto the flat from the channel and moved perpendicular, at the time, to the incoming current. On the relatively calm surface of the water, the school's wake looked like a moving, ribbed veil, some thirty feet across. The veil largely broke up as the fish slowed, broke ranks and began to hunt for prey, and then reformed as they picked up again, regrouped, and moved a short distance. They were getting comfortable and into a pattern, moving progressively closer to the skiff. I worried a little about a barracuda or bull shark entering the stage if I hooked-up, especially so close to the *Boca*, but I hadn't yet had even a single incident of double-predation, food-chain madness on this trip.

Now, with a little turn, the school was working directly up-current, straight for us, an easy cast away. I could see the individual fish now, each gray, torpedo shaped body and pointed snout reacting to any movement of escaping prey with a turn, a pause, and a resumption of forward movement with the school. *These Yucatán bonefish really move,* I observed. I decided to lead them more than I would a tailing, rooting fish. Right as the lead fish picked up again, my fly, a tried and true tan Mini-Puff, a number eight, turned over and touched down three or four feet in front of his nose, sending that satisfying drop of water an inch or two into the air. It touched bottom as the lead fish advanced to within a foot or so of it, and I stripped it in a little four-inch hop.

"Strip it, yes, that's good," Alfonso coached.

It wasn't necessary. When the fly touched bottom after the first strip, I saw the lead fish immediately leap forward, splay his pectorals as he braked and dipped down, and simultaneously felt my fly being sucked up, backwards, off the bottom and into the fish's mouth—it is a tactile game. At that same instant the fish turned ninety degrees and I struck him with a light pull on the fly line and a delicate side-sweep of the rod. The bonefish instantly reacted with a run and I loosened my grip on the departing fly line that had jumped to life at my feet, held it out to my side, and raised the rod tip. In a second the fish was on the little Ari T. Hart fly reel, which began to sing its uniquely pleasant song.

"M.G., get up here," I said.

And he was quickly at my shoulder to take the rod before the end of the first run.

I lay down on the middle bench to rest my back, and watched my friend play his first bonefish on a fly rod. Throughout the fish's many runs M.G. said, "I cannot believe the speed…," "He just won't stop…," "This freak of nature…," and "I refuse to believe a fish so small can run so far and so fast."

There is no better motivation. I smiled, knowing full well that he would now feel compelled to complete the transaction from start to finish. He would learn to cast, to spot them—these silver mirrors—through the water, to fool them with tufts of hair and feather, to play them well. He would want to know everything about them. Such is the nature of true addiction. I didn't know whether I was helping him or planting the seed of destruction in him. But it was inevitable, and with a friendship of thirty of our thirty-five years it was overdue.

I felt true happiness as I watched him unhook his first bonefish and get thoroughly slimed. I did not question this un-weighting of troubles my mind had just experienced through the simple act of giving away what is most cherished to me: the run of a bonefish.

I cast to and hooked up with another three bones, and gave the rod to my friend, who again said, "I'd be ashamed if it were anyone but you."

As the last fish was being released, my stomach suddenly went to water. I jumped onto the flat and quickly waded to the tapered drop off at channel's edge. M.G., as he let the last bonefish swim from his open hands, looked up and laughed at me.

I did not know it immediately, but I was bleeding profusely. The previous evening before going to bed, I had lost my balance in the tile shower stall while lathering my hair and blind, and fallen hard, hitting an edge with my tail rather than with my head. I had torn something, a small external tear, but also ruptured something internally. I believe the blood was mostly blood from the chronic dilation of my blood vessels in their reaction to the dedicated intake of alcohol, however. Booze is a powerful vasodilator that just relaxes most everything, including the muscles in one's arteries and veins. It's the same effect that results more benignly, over time, in that glowing, flush, burst-capillary nose of the drinker. This was the ugly side of it though, and I would learn that most of the alcoholics who do not die violently die by simply bleeding out through a vascular system so relaxed and opened up that they may as well have done it with a razor blade to the wrist (same thing, some would say).

So I lost a few ounces of blood, maybe a pint or more, and felt slightly weaker as I waded back to the skiff and, on my way, decided to forego the standard beer and eat a sandwich instead—that would surely help my energy. I was just gingerly sitting down on the skiff's bench, dripping salt water and not blood, reaching into the cooler for my sandwich when Alfonso said, "Look at the water, Jim."

I looked up to my guide and followed his eyes out over the flat, to the drop off where I'd just been. We now watched as two, seven to eight foot bull sharks were just arriving on the scene at breakneck speed. They began to dart around in classic agitation mode, hunting. Their fins were splayed erect at ninety degrees to the body, ready for quick maneuvering to snag evasive prey. I have never seen a pair of sharks more heated and "lit-up", ever. They were cutting and turning just down-tide of where I'd bled, hunting desperately for the source of the scent.

"They are looking for you, Jim," Alfonso quietly said. He stared at his client with a flat expression on his face, and slowly shook his head.

Guide's eyes, I thought. *He's seen the blood with those guide's eyes.* I shrugged my shoulders. I really did not think too much of the fact that two bull sharks had followed the panicked vibrations of four struggling bonefish to an extremely powerful source of scent. It made perfect sense, actually. *I'm out of harmony with the world, and am a part of the food chain as a result*, I thought to myself. I looked over to M.G. He was staring at me, his mouth hanging open in disbelief.

"I didn't see *that* in the brochure," he finally said.

I felt more shame at the prospect of my condition being found out than I did relief at not being at least attacked by sharks, if not consumed. I understood that, provided the right sequence of events occurs in this particular shark's presence, people are, indeed, on the menu. I had read of two Americans attacked and consumed off of Costa Rica by bull sharks a few years back, after their boat had been swamped outside of a river mouth while tarpon fishing. Deemed a negative for tourism, the attack was buried by the press, except for the obscure angling publication I had read. I had also personally witnessed this particular shark species behave shamelessly on more than one occasion because I had, by my very presence as an angler of warm salt waters, often set the dinner table for him and then rung the bell. It is the Zambeze shark of Africa, the Whaler of Australia, and the Lake Nicaragua shark of Central America—they are all the same shark:

the bull shark, _Carcharhinus leucas_. Leucas as in "Lucifer", to my mind. It is the one shark guilty of more attacks on man than all others. Combined.

In many warm regions of the world people do not actually have to go out of their way to mimic a natural prey item's behavior and be, therefore, "accidentally" attacked by this species of shark; this, for the simple fact that human beings _are_ a natural prey item for the bull shark. One theory is that, once exposed to mammals, bull sharks become "educated" ("addicted," perhaps?) and regularly consume them. All one must do to be accommodated is punch the right series of buttons, as I had just done. If one chose to do so, walking into the water under situations like I did would be analogous to "death by cop" in urban America, I felt, except with teeth rather than bullets. But unlike the good kind of cop who may find himself used as just such an instrument of death, the shark has no conscience and is just being a shark. This is what makes death by shark so impersonal and ghoulish: _Hey, do you even_ know _what you are eating, here?_

Watching the two sharks give up their hunt, I felt that one opportunity had just passed. "Not yet, I guess," I whispered to myself, as Alfonso put the boat on a plane. I realized this is what the dying must say: _Not yet._ Rather than a heated rush of panic, I felt a simple hunger. I ate the last lobster sandwich, sans beer. "Spiny lobster kicks Maine lobster's ass," I said to M.G., who, still processing the scene, merely nodded.

* * *

Alfonso poled the skiff parallel to a long key on the west side of the lagoon, hugging an edge where white sand met dark green turtle grass; the wind, angled into our shoulders and backs, was now up to twenty miles per hour or so, and thin clouds were scudding by quickly overhead.

"Behind you," Alfonso said. "Two permit—too fast."

I turned around and looked behind the boat where two permit were coming out of five o'clock, seventy or eighty feet away, and moving too fast to spin the boat for an easier shot.

They made little if any wake, as they were swimming with the wind this time, out of the east; but I saw their whole black-topped, silver bodies as they came off of the dark turtle grass onto the open white sand. My eye locked on the lead, target fish; I roll cast Alfonso's crab fly out of my fingers, out over the water and, while I could cast through the boat from bow to stern, there was no time to tell everyone to duck and there was still that push pole in Alfonso's hands, so I raised the rod handle up to my head to give the cast plenty of height, and held it off my opposite shoulder to clear the boat. It was restricted, but this rod and line were extensions of my body and, after one complete false cast, I had the belly of the fly line out of the rod tip in the air behind me and I shot a little more, locked it down and came forward, hit it with a push of the thumb, the moderate power all aimed at a spot about six feet in front of the approaching fish, and let the cast go. There was a lovely zip-song as the friction-reducing bumps on the stiff running line shot through the rod guides, and then an almost audible splat as the fat fly hit the target area.

"Gooood," Alfonso whispered. "Let it sink…Now strip it, strip it— keep stripping it, Jim."

I felt out of body, as if I were no longer a physical entity, but a slowed sequence of events in time, in this specific space, instead. Fly line, tippet, water, moving fish, moving fly. I made myself the fly in the water. I heeded Alfonso's advice without hesitation, without question. I accepted that Mexican permit must eat swimming crab flies because there must be lots of swimming crabs in Mexico. I kept stripping it and by now the lead-eyed fly was angling up near the surface, and I witnessed the lead permit as she rose with the fly, hot in pursuit, her schoolmate staying in wing man position and not trying to overtake her and her perceived grail. Then I saw, as they were propelled above the water's surface: the permit's graceful, long black dorsal fin and the tip of her caudal fin, her back and almost half of her head, and then finally her huge orb of an eye—yes, her eye—about to break the surface of the water, intently focused on the fly at the surface. And this fish of noble blood, now cross-eyed like a cartoon caricature of herself, desperately inhaled the fly which I had not stopped moving, submerged with it and turned. I felt her resistance and struck her with the tight line in my line hand and a sweep of the powerful ten weight into its mid section. She immediately reacted by bolting off at blazing velocity, and the fly line at my feet danced into the air, off the deck as it sped to meet the rod guides. She was headed for open water, which was safest, and I raised the rod up and away, tilting the reel outward, and held the retreating fly line out to my other side with lightly pinched thumb, index and middle finger pressure. She got onto the reel in a smooth transition and continued running, water dancing in a white razor streak along the departing fly line, and my Hart S2 fell into its defined song on the speedy and steady out-take of line and now, backing. I finally exhaled an aged breath.

"Permit came out of the water to eat your fly," Alfonso said, shaking his head and smiling. "Never see that before."

"Are there any sharks around?" I asked.

"No," Alfonso said, and then laughed.

The permit made several steady, fifty to hundred yard runs, and then the close-in struggle began. She turned her broad sides to me throughout. I was a little light on this fish, not pushing it, worried about the hook loosing. Some ten minutes after hook-up, with a slowed run towards the rear of the boat, I used her forward motion and guided the fish with nose-lifting pressure towards Alfonso, who was standing in the bilge, and the fish was tired enough this time that the deftly sweeping Mayan arm found its mark and tailed the permit perfectly, the guide's fist encircling the tight caudal peduncle that trademarks only the most powerful families of fish in the world, the tunas, bill fish, mackeral sharks and the jacks, the Carangids, to which family the permit belongs. A beaming Alfonso lifted her gently into the air: a bona fide permit of around six or seven pounds in weight.

"Your first permit, Mr. Jim," he said, walking with the fish towards me, one hand under her little belly for support, just in front of that unique and colorful ventral splash of yellow. "And for me, she is the very first permit to eat a dry fly."

Water was streaming down her silver body as I gently put my rod down and took her. She is truly a pretty fish, the permit; and the heart of this beauty which the human searches for in all creatures—something tangible that reflects shared life experience and travail—I found in her clear, liquid, silver-dollar-sized eyes. I took my sunglasses off and looked into her eye, the obsidian pupil of which was staring transfixed down into the water—live fish always stare into the water if they can see it, I remembered. She did not meet my gaze, but continued to look into the water and work her rubbery mouth in the suffocating air, beseeching me, *put me back.*

Properly realized, she is the pinnacle of achievement, the permit.

As I held her, I thought of Islamorada, a decade ago: "Your cast is technically perfect," Captain Ruoff, a kind mentor, had said to me. And the air had suddenly parted with a whisk of breeze then, as a flight of introduced, yet now generations very much wild, green parrots dipped down low at breakneck speed, right over our heads to check us out, and then rose gradually back up, higher, and continued on towards a mangrove hummock where they lighted to roost . "Live well, Jim," Rick had said, on parting.

Holding my first permit, I laughed. *I am a technically perfect mess.* Rick knew when he'd said it, anyway, that perfect and "pretty" casters are regularly destroyed on the flats by high winds and other adverse conditions. I had evolved into a reaction-caster, a predator. I felt my teacher would be proud of that. But only that.

I looked into the permit's black, incorruptible eye. I felt unworthy of her, and a prickly and troubled warmth, a confused rush, rose in my chest. But here she was, in my hands. *Yes, honest skill has earned her—mine and Alfonso's.* Holding this Holy Grail of saltwater angling, I knew that any arm chair psychologist would say I had finally caught myself. I would rather listen to the fish. I looked at my reflection in the liquid, mirrored blackness of the permit's pupil, saw the reconstructed face. *That's not me. I am nothing.*

The permit moved her huge orb of an eye in its socket to look up at my face, and then turned to look back down to the water. "Oh. Sorry," I said to the permit.

M.G. and Alfonso were watching me, beginning to appear concerned.

I lay down on my chest on the platform and put the permit back in the water. She lightly kicked. I gently held her lower jaw open half-way with my thumb and, clasping her tail juncture, I pushed her slowly back and forth in the water until she undulated more firmly. I let her swim off.

I never took my eye off her as I washed my hands with sand from the bottom and watched as my first permit, a cast away, slowly ghosted over the white sand, turned, and swam back into the green turtle grass forest, where she disappeared.

Tens of millions of years ago meteors smashed into the earth not far from here and time stopped forever for much of life. Time stopped again for a moment, just for me.

"Thank you," I said to my fish, the water and the sea grass. I turned to look at M.G. "How about another bonefish?"

"Absolutely," he said.

Alfonso was nodding his head, too, and smiling.

"I might want to try and cast a fly to them this time, too—if that's okay," M.G. added.

"God help us," I said.

"I think he just did, Jimbo, " M.G. said.

You're a perceptive man, M.G., I thought to myself.

"Yup," I said. "And asking His help with your casting would be asking way too much," I said.

* * *

August 2004, West Galveston Bay, Texas, USA.

It was all simple after releasing the permit: I picked a date for a qualified medical detoxification from alcohol and stuck with it. I was informed that, as much as I drank, I would have died of an alcohol withdrawl seizure without the medical assistance.

I have not drunk alcohol since, and this fine day I am standing on the casting platform of my staked-off Mitzi skiff—named the *Miniscus* on a good day, and the *Bone-R* on a bad day—in a sea grass bottomed cove in my home waters of Texas as a result of this simple fact.

If I have boat trouble most anywhere I like to fish in this bay, I can indeed, by God, step out of the skiff into the water and simply walk home, as the great John D. McDonald observed of Keys waters in his Travis McGee classics. Of August it is truly "the doldrums", as there isn't even a hint of a breeze to cool me or to riffle the water's surface and calm the fish. I notice that there is no singing or nagging from the usual complement of wading birds, gulls and terns. There is no sound, in fact, unless I decide to make some, and it feels dulled, muted, as if I am in a vacuum of dead space.

I cast a weedless fly, my *Sin Ensalada* ("no salad", in Spanish), with my eight weight fly rod, targeting the random tan sand spots, ridges and channels that contrast starkly against the massive expanse of green *Halodule* eel grass that carpets the bottom. Seatrout and redfish love these little oases in the dense forest. They ambush baitfish, shrimp and crabs that find their way into these spots and become, quite suddenly, obvious prey spotlighted on the stage. My rod is loaded with a nearly transparent floating fly line that allows me to "line" a lot of fish I may not see without them always being aware of the insult. When covering likely fish territory and not exclusively sight-fishing, I am convinced that the clear floating line, a Monic made by Bob Goodale in Colorado, more than doubles the number of fish I catch on any given day. This more random method of casting a fly also allows me to relax between sight-castings to targeted fish. And relaxing, while not my initial or intended goal, has become a casual side effect of a new way of life.

After I have fished the fly a ways down a defined edge of a sandy lane, my eye catches a turning flash of amber red, right about where my fly should be. Simultaneously I feel the fly line stop to firm resistance, and I react with a sharp pull on the line and a quick whip of the rod to the side. A bulge of water appears above the redfish as she thrashes and then kicks away on her first run, pulling the stripped-out fly line off the deck through my lightly clasping left hand. She's quickly onto the little Hart fly reel and running slowly but steadily straight out, which is characteristic of a more sizable red. I wonder, again, what would happen if I were to tie a five pound redfish tail-to-tail to a five pound bonefish. I rarely think such thoughts while I am in the middle of playing one or the other and lost in the enjoyment, but I am today because I will be bonefishing again soon, for Ascension Bay fish.

"Boy, that would be one big argument, too," I say to myself. I remember fishing the Upper Cross Banks in Florida Bay where the innumerable three foot bonnethead sharks always hunt at the top of the flat in the mangrove shoots, their dorsal and caudal fins waving in the air as they course along, and where bonefish and redfish are reputed to hunt side by side. I have caught silvery redfish there with my friend, Captain Rick Miller, and I hope to at least see the other species there when I return. There is something comforting in the idea of these two fine game fish coexisting in some areas, crossing paths and bidding each other, "Hello. Why, yes—the crabs are excellent today."

I catch myself in drifting thoughts again, and remind myself that I must stay focused. "I'm insulting a perfectly good redfish by thinking about bonefish, and other things," I say to myself.

This redfish looks really red in color through the water, I notice, over the green sea grass—it's like Christmas. When she's out of the water, in my hands, however, she appears more of an amber color dorsally, with almost silver sides. *It must be the way the light refracts in the water.* Her neon blue-tipped tail glows in the sunshine, as if it were one big, fiery, baby blue Light Emitting Diode.

Her eyes are staring into the water, so I pop the de-barbed fly out with my thumb pushing down and backwards at the eye. After I release the fish over the gunwale and rise up to my knees, I look up and see in the sky a coiled gray snake of cloud working down from the thunderhead a mile or so to the north. It is a waterspout, and a big one. I see white spray rise in a bloom where the funnel's apex touches the water's surface. But here where I stand the air is completely still and there is no sound but the blood pulsing regularly and calmly in my ears.

Of course this thunderhead is not stationary, but is moving slowly to the south, towards me. I have time, though, about fifteen minutes, to safely watch as the spout either continues on its general course, or doesn't. Either way I will have to move, as this is a big wall of thunderheads, and where there's one spout there can form another. I get the camera, snap a few shots, and wish for a zoom lens. *Soon I won't need a zoom lens,* I realize. *It's time to go.* I sit on the cockpit seat and put the camera back into the dry bag, reach around to untie the push pole from the poling platform, and just then I see the spout lift from the water and quickly dissolve in the air as its generating forces die and its remnants are sucked back up into the thunderhead. A benign, light breeze is born. The birds relax, and I hear the first nasal snorts from a pod of white ibis hidden behind some wind-swept live oaks, and the growing cackle of laughing gulls as they take to the air again. Things appear to be back to normal. I pick up the eight weight fly rod, and fish.

From the bow platform I look to the shoreline and see a large push of water and a high, triangular dorsal fin some two feet behind it, paralleling the shore, some two hundred feet from my boat. I look into the water at the bulge and see a long, brown, linebacker-sized, fluidly swimming form that is of flexible cartilage, and can only be one thing in these waters: a substantial and, at present, relaxed bull shark. There have been a great number of them in the bay this summer, and a few sober fishermen I know have been reporting incidents of double-predation by the sharks, the predators taking full advantage of a banner season of hooked redfish and trout. And Dr. Landry, my former Ichthyology professor, had just recently corroborated these incidents and sightings of <u>Carcharhinus leucas</u> on the local news, which gave a sense of vindication to me: the local recovering alcoholic fishing population was not, indeed, off the wagon and imagining things.

The placid shark reaches a widely spaced line of old wood and newer PVC stakes perpendicular to the shoreline, and casually turns to follow them out, directly towards my skiff. Approaching head on, I see the great blunt width of the shark's snout, a defining trait of the bull. This fish's mouth is as broad as a man's waist. I had been wading in this very spot yesterday and had drawn a smaller shark in close by hooking up, playing, and releasing a pair of nice redfish. He had homed in on and followed the last red to within a hundred feet of me. Now I felt sure that that fish, also, was a bull. *And because I was not bleeding into the water at the time, the shark simply swam away when it knew a man was in the water with him.*

Today, I watch the shark as it swims towards me, so strikingly fluid with his whole body involved in it, unknowing of my very presence. I smile. This shark must be doing exactly what I'm doing: *he's redfishing.* Or, *I've heard they eat stingrays, which are all over this huge flat all the time. I bet he's redfishing today, like me.*

Realizing it would be pointless to cast a #4 redfish fly on eight pound tippet to a three to five hundred pound shark, I decide to put down my fly rod and get the camera, which is back in the dry bag, in the seat compartment, to take a picture of the shark. I cannot quite believe something so large is in such shallow water, as I always think when I see such things, even though the fish is right here, some fifty feet away by now. I move as cautiously as I can, slowly lowering the fly rod behind me; but as the cork butt of it touches the bottom of the cockpit, the mass of the steel and aluminum fly reel rotates the rod downward with gravity, and taps the fiberglass hull in an audible "tap".

"Oops," I whisper, cringing.

All I can do is watch. It has been a long time since I've seen anything so large move so fast. All that belies the shark's former presence in the cove is a flowering plume of gray-brown sand suspended in the clear water, a concave hole on its surface, and a blazing, departing ridge of brine that reflects mirrored silver under the sun. Everything is suddenly still again. A moment later the wake from the shark reaches my skiff and gently rocks it. The birds begin to sing again.

I am outside of the pain.

The cycle has been broken, and another begins anew. It is one of only two life cycles a human being can live: a benign circle, or a malignant, vicious circle. One feeds and nourishes itself, and also those of others, while the other consumes and destroys itself and others. Either cycle can be broken.

Many believe that if something is meant to be, it will happen. This may be true for some, especially lazy types. For others, however, with all things of any significance, if they are meant to be we must *make* them happen. I trust noble efforts are not lost to God, and are rewarded in kind. Sometimes even on earth.

Whom God would save
He first makes a bonefisherman.

* * *

BIBLIOGRAPHY

1.) Reiger, George, ed., <u>The Bonefish</u>, Meadow Run Press, Stone Harbor, New Jersey, 1993, pp. 100-117.
2.) Cole, John, <u>Tarpon Quest</u>, Lyons and Burford, New York, New York, 1991, p.50.
3.) Bond, Carl E., <u>Biology of Fishes</u>, Holt, Rinehart and Winston, Orlando, Florida, 1979, pp. 148-149.
4.) Cardenas, Jeffrey, <u>Marquesa</u>, Meadow Run Press, Stone Harbor, New Jersey, 1995, pp. 24-25.

ORGANIZATIONS

Tarpon and Bonefish Unlimited, respectively, can be accessed via the internet at:

www.tarbone.org

The Coastal Conservation Association, headquartered nationally in Houston, Texas, can be reached via internet at: www.joincca.org

ABOUT THE AUTHOR

A native Texan and direct descendant of founding families of Texas, Jim was Certified nationally in 1994 as a casting instructor by James "Chi-co" Fernandez and Lefty Kreh of the Federation of Fly Fishers. A former Texas fly fishing columnist, Jim lives on Galveston Island's West End, in Houston, and in the Texas Hill Country.

www.ingramcontent.com/pod-product-compliance
Lightning Source LLC
Chambersburg PA
CBHW030401290526
45785CB00004B/1851